Albert A. Herzog, Jr., PhD, MDiv, MA
Editor

Disability Advocacy Among Religious Organizations: Histories and Reflections

Disability Advocacy Among Religious Organizations: Histories and Reflections has been co-published simultaneously as *Journal of Religion, Disability & Health*, Volume 10, Numbers 1/2 2006.

Pre-publication REVIEWS, COMMENTARIES, EVALUATIONS . . .

" A N ABSOLUTE "MUST HAVE" for all seminary libraries and for agencies and individuals seeking to work for and with persons with disabilities today."

William H. Swatos, Jr., PhD, MA, MDiv
Executive Officer, Religious Research Organization, Executive Officer, Association for the Sociology of Religion, Senior Fellow, Center for Religious Inquiry Across the Disciplines (CRIAD), Baylor University, Editor-in-Chief, Encyclopedia of Religion and Society

D0165432

Disability Advocacy Among Religious Organizations: Histories and Reflections

Disability Advocacy Among Religious Organizations: Histories and Reflections has been co-published simultaneously as *Journal of Religion, Disability & Health*, Volume 10, Numbers 1/2 2006.

Monographic Separates from the *Journal of Religion, Disability & Health*

For additional information on these and other Haworth Press titles, including descriptions, tables of contents, reviews, and prices, use the QuickSearch catalog at http://www.HaworthPress.com.

Disability Advocacy Among Religious Organizations: Histories and Reflections edited by Albert A. Herzog, J., PhD, MDiv, MA (Vol. 10, No. 1/2, 2006). *Insightful exploration of the histories of disability advocacy within numerous religious organizations since 1950.*

End-of-Life Care: Bridging Disability and Aging with Person-Centered Care, edited by Rev. William C. Gaventa, MDiv, and David L. Coulter, MD (Vol. 9, No. 2, 2005). *A probing set of examinations into disability, Alzheimer's, and end-of-life debates, using a pair of cogent arguments as a starting point, followed by carefully considered responses from other experts.*

Critical Reflections on Stanley Hauerwas' Theology of Disability: Disabling Society, Enabling Theology, edited by John Swinton, PhD (Vol. 8, No. 3/4, 2004). *"AN EXCELLENT AND LONG-NEEDED RESOURCE. . . . This work will not only continue the ongoing discussion among those specializing in the theology of disability in general and disability related to intellectual development in particular, but will also serve to bring disability into the mainline of contemporary theological discussion." (Kerry H. Wynn, PhD, Director, Learning Enrichment Center, Southeast Missouri State University)*

Voices in Disability and Spirituality from the Land Down Under: From Outback to Outfront, edited by Rev. Dr. Christopher Newell, PhD, and Rev. Andy Calder (Vol. 8, No. 1/2, 2004). *"In recent years disability theology has emerged alongside Black theology and womens' theology as a new genre seeking to express the concerns of people whose experience has often been marginalized. This collection is A SIGNIFICANT AUSTRALIAN CONTRIBUTION TO THIS GROWING LITERATURE. The early explorers named Australia 'the south land of the Holy Spirit.' (John M. Hull, PhD, Hon DTheol, Professor Emeritus of Religious Education, University of Birmingham, England; Author of* On Sight and Insight *and* In the Beginning There Was Darkness).

Graduate Theological Education and the Human Experience of Disability, edited by Robert C. Anderson (Vol. 7, No. 3, 2003). *"A comprehensive overview of theological education and disability. . . . Concise and well written. . . . Offers rich theological insights and abundant practical advice. I strongly recommend this volume as a key introduction to this important emerging topic in theological education." (Rev. John W. Crossin, PhD, OSFS, Executive Director, Washington Theological Consortium)*

The Pastoral Voice of Robert Perske, edited by William C. Gaventa, Jr., MDiv, and David L. Coulter, MD (Vol. 7, No. 1/2, 2003). *"Must reading for seminary students and clininical program directors. Pastors, providers, and parents concerned with persons suffering from cognitive, intellectual, and developmental disabilities will find these vigorous testimonies readable, timely, fresh, and inspiring despite having been written more than 30 years ago." (Barbara J. Lampe, JD, Executive Director, National Apostolate for Inclusion Ministry)*

Spirituality and Intellectual Disability: International Perspectives on the Effect of Culture and Religion on Healing Body, Mind, and Soul, edited by William C. Gaventa, Jr., MDiv, and David L. Coulter, MD (Vol. 5, No. 2/3, 2001). *"Must reading . . . perspectives from many faiths and cultures on the spiritual needs and gifts of people with mental retardation." (Ginny Thornburgh, EdM, Religion and Disability Program, National Organization on Disability, Washington, DC)*

The Theological Voice of Wolf Wolfensberger, edited by William C. Gaventa, MDiv, and David L. Coulter, MD (Vol. 4, No. 2/3, 2001). *This thought-provoking volume presents Wolfensberger's challenging, outrageous, and inspiring ideas on the theological significance of disabilities, including the problem with wheelchair access ramps in churches, the meaning of suffering, and the spiritual gifts of the mentally retarded.*

Disability Advocacy Among Religious Organizations: Histories and Reflections

Albert A. Herzog, Jr., PhD, MDiv, MA
Editor

Disability Advocacy Among Religious Organizations: Histories and Reflections has been co-published simultaneously as *Journal of Religion, Disability & Health*, Volume 10, Numbers 1/2 2006.

The Haworth Pastoral Press®
An Imprint of The Haworth Press, Inc.

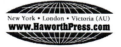

New York • London • Victoria (AU)
www.HaworthPress.com

Published by

The Haworth Pastoral Press®, 10 Alice Street, Binghamton, NY 13904-1580 USA

The Haworth Pastoral Press® is an imprint of The Haworth Press, Inc., 10 Alice Street, Binghamton, NY 13904-1580 USA.

Disability Advocacy Among Religious Organizations: Histories and Reflections has been co-published simultaneously as *Journal of Religion, Disability & Health,* Volume 10, Numbers 1/2 2006.

Cover design by Lora Wiggins

Library of Congress Cataloging-in-Publication Data

Disability advocacy among religious organizations : histories and reflections / Albert A. Herzog, Jr., editor.
    p. cm.
    "Co-published simultaneously as Journal of religion, disability & health, Volume 10, numbers 1/2 2006."–P.
    Includes bibliographical references and index.
    ISBN–13: 978-0-7890-3289-8 (hard cover : alk. paper)
    ISBN–10: 0-7890-3289-9 (hard cover : alk. paper)
    ISBN–13: 978-0-7890-3290-4 (soft cover : alk. paper)
    ISBN–10: 0-7890-3290-2 (soft cover : alk. paper)
    1. Church work with people with disabilities. 2. Legal assistance to people with disabilities. I. Herzog, Albert A., 1944-.
  BV4460.D57 2006
  261.8'324–dc22   2005037767

Indexing, Abstracting & Website/Internet Coverage

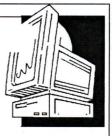

This section provides you with a list of major indexing & abstracting services and other tools for bibliographic access. That is to say, each service began covering this periodical during the year noted in the right column. Most Websites which are listed below have indicated that they will either post, disseminate, compile, archive, cite or alert their own Website users with research-based content from this work. (This list is as current as the copyright date of this publication.)

Abstracting, Website/Indexing Coverage . . . . Year When Coverage Began

- *Applied Social Sciences Index & Abstracts (ASSIA)*
  (Online: ASSI via Data-Star) (CDRom: ASSIA Plus)
  <http://www.csa.com> . . . . *
- *AURSI African Urban & Regional Science Index. A scholarly &*
  research index which synthesises & compiles all publications
  on urbanization & regional science in Africa within the world.
  Published annually **2004**
- *CINAHL (Cumulative Index to Nursing & Allied Health*
  Literature), in print, EBSCO, and SilverPlatter, DataStar,
  and PaperChase (Support materials include Subject Heading List,
  Database Search Guide, and instructional video)
  <http://www.cinahl.com> **1999**
- *e-psyche, LLC <http://www.e-psyche.net>* . . . . *
- *EBSCOhost Electronic Journals Service (EJS)*
  <http://ejournals.ebsco.com> **2001**
- *Educational Research Abstracts (ERA) (online database)*
  <http://www.tandf.co.uk/era> **2003**
- *Elsevier Scopus <http://www.info.scopus.com>* **2005**
- *Family & Society Studies Worldwide*
  <http://www.nisc.com> . . . . *
- *Family Index Database <http://www.familyscholar.com>* **2003**
- *Google <http://www.google.com>* **2004**
- *Google Scholar <http://scholar.google.com>* **2004**
- *Haworth Document Delivery Center*
  <http://www.HaworthPress.com/journals/dds.asp> **1999**
- *Human Resources Abstracts (HRA)* . . . . *

(continued)

Special Bibliographic Notes related to special journal issues (separates) and indexing/abstracting:

- indexing/abstracting services in this list will also cover material in any "separate" that is co-published simultaneously with Haworth's special thematic journal issue or DocuSerial. Indexing/abstracting usually covers material at the article/chapter level.
- monographic co-editions are intended for either non-subscribers or libraries which intend to purchase a second copy for their circulating collections.
- monographic co-editions are reported to all jobbers/wholesalers/approval plans. The source journal is listed as the "series" to assist the prevention of duplicate purchasing in the same manner utilized for books-in-series.
- to facilitate user/access services all indexing/abstracting services are encouraged to utilize the co-indexing entry note indicated at the bottom of the first page of each article/chapter/contribution.
- this is intended to assist a library user of any reference tool (whether print, electronic, online, or CD-ROM) to locate the monographic version if the library has purchased this version but not a subscription to the source journal.
- individual articles/chapters in any Haworth publication are also available through the Haworth Document Delivery Service (HDDS).

Disability Advocacy
Among Religious Organizations:
Histories and Reflections

CONTENTS

ABOUT THE EDITOR

Albert A. Herzog, Jr., PhD, MDiv, MA, received his PhD from the Ohio State University and is a full-time Lecturer in Sociology at the Ohio State University, Newark Campus. After writing a dissertation on religion and politics, Dr. Herzog worked as a researcher for the National Science Foundation, the United Methodist Church and the Ohio Department of Health. In recent years, his research and presentations at professional meetings has focused on the relationship between religion and disability with several papers on the disability ministries of mainline denominations and the National Council of Churches. The research for some of these works have been funded by the Louisville Institute and the Religious Research Association. He is an ordained Elder in the United Methodist Church.

Introduction:
Disability Advocacy
Among Religious Organizations

Albert A. Herzog, Jr., PhD, MDiv, MA

The articles in this combined collection provide histories of disability advocacy among religious organizations, especially since 1950. As such, they are but brief glimpses into the past as to how disability advocacy became a part of their respective organizations, how their program was shaped and with what emphases, what was accomplished, and how they are currently positioned with respect to disability advocacy–both in terms of their social location within the religious organization and the larger social arena of other religious organizations and the society at large.

From the point of view of religious history, it appears appropriate to state that as the history of religious organizations is told, disability advocacy should be told also. And while disability advocacy "should" or "ought" to be told alongside other stories (as, for example, women and various other groups), disability-related topics are rarely, if ever, broached. Nevertheless, disability advocacy among religious organizations is a story that not only *should* be told, but *can* be told because there are documents available from numerous sources, people from the past who are still around to tell their stories, and live, active groups, still at the work of disability advocacy whose presence bares witness to past efforts.

[Haworth co-indexing entry note]: "Introduction: Disability Advocacy Among Religious Organiza-tions." Herzog, Albert A. Jr. Co-published simultaneously in *Journal of Religion, Disability & Health* (The Haworth Pastoral Press, an imprint of The Haworth Press, Inc.) Vol. 10, No. 1/2, 2006, pp. 1-3; and: *Disability Advocacy Among Religious Organizations: Histories and Reflections* (ed: Albert A. Herzog, Jr.) The Haworth Pastoral Press, an imprint of The Haworth Press, Inc., 2006, pp. 1-3. Single or multiple copies of this article are available for a fee from The Haworth Document Delivery Service [1-800-HAWORTH, 9:00 a.m. - 5:00 p.m. (EST). E-mail address: docdelivery@haworthpress.com].

doi:10.1300/J095v10n01_01

While I am sure that Catherine Albanese's (Albanese, 1981:1) appropriation of the story told by some Buddhists and Muslims about "blind men" trying to describe the elephant will raise the eyebrows of some readers, her slant on "the elephant in the dark" is true. Religious life has many dimensions and "nobody ever will know the whole story because the vastness that surrounds us far exceeds our senses or our ability to understand."

Yet, there is also the sense that the stories in the articles which follow need to be told because disability history has become an important topic on the contemporary scene with respect to the academic study of disability. This is indicated by the emergence of a historiography of disability (see Longmore and Umansky, 2001), the establishment of the Disability History Association (Burch, 2005), and the emergence of disability paper sessions and efforts at "embracing disability in teaching religion" by the American Academy of Religion (Wynn, 2005). In addition, it is of no small consequence that the Society for Disability Studies will devote its Summer, 2006 issue of *Disability Studies Quarterly* to the theme, "Religious, Spirituality, and Disability Studies" (Society for Disability Studies, 2005).

How then can the articles which follow be placed into this context? To start, when this special edition was contemplated, we (Bill Gaventa and I) asked leaders in religious organizations doing disability advocacy to submit, in article form, a history of their work since 1950. Specifically, we asked each writer to: (1) provide a summary of any history prior to 1950; (2) summarize developments focusing on major accomplishments, strategies that worked, relationships with secular movements and other issues since 1950; (3) indicate "model practices" of ministries within the religious organization since 1950; and (4) anticipated directions in the future.

These articles provide a start to uncovering and analyzing disability advocacy among religious organizations. It is my conviction that they should be allowed to "tell their own story" and thus their authors to "speak for themselves." I hope that they will provide for those of us who are "in the field" a new awareness that "we are not alone" and that there is a reservoir of ideas no single program of disability advocacy would ever be able to employ. It is also my hope that disability studies scholars and church historians will see the value of the study of disability advocacy as an important segment in evaluating religious responses to disability and to social issues in general.

REFERENCES

Albanese, C. L. (1981). *America: Religions and Religion*. Belmont, CA: Wadsworth.

Burch, S. (2005). *Join the Disability History Association*. Retrieved from: Society for Disability Studies, July 7, 2005 (SDS_Listerv@LISTSERV.UIC.edu).

Kirchner, C. (2005). *Disability Studies Quarterly, Summer 2006, Theme Issues "Religious, Spirituality, and Disability Studies"–Call for Abstracts*. Retrieved from: Society for Disability Studies, August 19, 2005 (SDS_Listerv@LISTSERV.UIC.edu).

Longmore, P.K., & L. Umansky (Eds.) (2001) *The New Disability History: American Perspectives*. New York: New York University Press.

Wynn, K. (Ed.) (2005). *Embracing Disability in Teaching Religion, Spotlight on Teaching*. Atlanta: American Academy of Religion.

The Ecumenical Response to Disability: The World Council of Churches

Sam Kabue

SUMMARY. Since the late 1960s, disability issues have been on the agenda of the World Council of Churches. Emerging from its Faith Order Commission as a theological examination of disability in light of the compassion of Christ, the various forms of action have raised the conscience of member communions and the WCC organization. The ministry has taken many forms depending on financial and other resources. Its most recent forum, EDAN (Ecumenical Disability Advocates Network) has held consultations around the globe and has developed an interim theological statement "A Church of All and For All." *[Article copies available for a fee from The Haworth Document Delivery Service: 1-800-HAWORTH. E-mail address: <docdelivery@haworthpress.com> Website: <http://www.HaworthPress.com> © 2006 by The Haworth Press, Inc. All rights reserved.]*

KEYWORDS. World Council of Churches, disability, EDAN, A Church of All and For All

The Ecumenical movement has in the last thirty years or so found itself faced with the necessity of addressing disability as a concern. After the fourth Assembly of the World Council of Churches in 1968, the

---

Sam Kabue is the Coordinator for Ecumenical Disability Advocacy Network, World Council of Churches working out of the All Africa Council of Churches in Nairobi, Kenya. He has a background in education and recreation, and has served as a representative from Kenya to United Nations organizations concerning disability issues.

[Haworth co-indexing entry note]: "The Ecumenical Response to Disability: The World Council of Churches." Kabue, Sam. Co-published simultaneously in *Journal of Religion, Disability & Health* (The Haworth Pastoral Press, an imprint of The Haworth Press, Inc.) Vol. 10, No. 1/2, 2006, pp. 5-10; and: *Disability Advocacy Among Religious Organizations: Histories and Reflections* (ed: Albert A. Herzog, Jr.) The Haworth Pastoral Press, an imprint of The Haworth Press, Inc., 2006, pp. 5-10. Single or multiple copies of this article are available for a fee from The Haworth Document Delivery Service [1-800-HAWORTH, 9:00 a.m. - 5:00 p.m. (EST). E-mail address: docdelivery@haworthpress.com].

Available online at http://www.haworthpress.com/web/JRDH
doi:10.1300/J095v10n01_02

theme "The Unity of the Church and the Renewal of Humankind" emerged as a means of relating issues of church and society. At the Assembly and subsequently, the attempt to explore the church as a more inclusive community intensified. A concern to address the inclusion of people with disabilities in the church emerged within the Faith and Order Commission, and gathered momentum at the Louvain meeting of the Commission in 1971. This first attempt to address the situation of persons with disabilities was a theological examination of service for the disabled in the light of the compassion of Christ.

WCC has thus since the Faith and order Commission Louvain 1971 meeting incorporated persons with disabilities in its wider mission and agenda. Effort has been made to include them and to advocate for their recognition in the member churches. In the 1975, WCC General Assembly in Nairobi, Kenya the Council reiterated its commitment to the concerns of persons with disabilities through a statement which sought to mobilize the member churches to make similar commitments. The emphasis during this time was on the services and programs that the Council and member churches could put in place in favor of people with disabilities.

In 1977, a staff Task Force on Persons with Disabilities was established to help take further the ideas that had been agreed on in the previous Assembly. Two consultations were organized for this purpose which considered various aspects of disability in Bad Saarow, Germany in 1978 and in Sao Paul, Brazil thereafter. From 1978 onwards, the Christian Medical Commission held a series of seven regional conferences on the theme: "Health, Healing, and Wholeness."

A full-time consultant, Ms. Frances Martin, was appointed in 1980 for eighteen months to help the Task Force concientise the churches during the United Nations International Year of Disabled Persons. At the WCC Six Assembly, in Vancouver, Canada in 1983, there were 21 persons with disabilities, the largest participation in any assembly before. Deliberations in the Assembly reiterated the need for the churches to accommodate disability concerns in their life and ministry.

In affirming the above, the Council established a disability desk with a full-time member of the staff in Geneva in 1984. A lot of work in sensitizing churches was carried out for the next seven years. Contacts were re-established with member churches, national and regional ecumenical bodies, church and secular agencies working with persons with disabilities. Unfortunately, the staff was discontinued in 1991 because of lack of funds. For the next three years, the work was carried out by a Task Force until 1994 when another member of staff was hired on consultancy basis. Taking over from the Task Force and with their assistance, the new member of staff was responsible for this work until 1996 when the position was again discontinued. Thus, the Task Force took up the work as the Council prepared to go to its 8th Assembly. One of the most remarkable achievements of the Task Force at that time was the 1997 Central Committee statement to the churches. That theological and sociological statement was the first document that was sent out to all the churches to urge them to consider the question of active involvement of persons with disabilities as part of the churches. The Task Force worked with that statement to ensure participation of persons with disabilities in the 8th WCC General Assembly in Harare, Zimbabwe in 1998.

WCC, however, was seeking new ways of carrying out this work at minimum expenses and maximum efficiency without necessarily having to establish an expensive structure in Geneva. Their vision was to decentralize their work by passing responsibility on certain aspects to other partners with capacity and willingness to carry it out. During the WCC 8th Assembly, 10 persons with disabilities from different parts of the world were invited to participate as advisors. In their role as advisors they took the opportunity to hold their own consultations as to how best to influence the churches to recognize and incorporate people with disabilities in their witness and service program.

The 10 advisors decided to form a network known as Ecumenical Disability Advocates Network (EDAN) that would carry the WCC work on disability further to respective regions where each individual came from. EDAN as a network and initiative of persons with disabilities was considered by WCC a model idea for work with persons with disabilities. WCC proposed to support the work through an ecumenical partner with both the interest and the working structure necessary for this kind of work. NCCK was identified as a suitable host as it was one of the councils that was already doing some work in this respect.

EDAN is therefore a WCC programme and is situated within the Justice, Peace and Creation (JPC) team. Its placement in this team is significant as an acknowledgement that WCC recognizes disability concerns as justice issues. The Network carries out its work in various regions using the WCC regional structures. Its mandate is to advocate for inclusion, participation and observation of rights of persons with disabilities through networks allied to these structures.

A WCC Interim Theological Statement was the product of close to three years process of consultations and discussions under EDAN with the assistance and guidance of Faith and Order. This new interim statement, "A Church of All and For All," is thus a stage on a continuing journey. In developing it, we have benefited from very helpful contributions by a group of disabled individuals–many of whom are ordained ministers or students of theology–and by parents of disabled children and by others who experience life alongside people with disabilities in various ways. It is an invitation to the churches to journey with us toward that radical place where all are welcomed at God's banquet table.

The statement is not a comprehensive document but offers pointers and insights on major theological themes. It has very distinct sections on the commonalities and differences, the hermeneutical issue, Imago Dei, Healing, and Forgiveness, Giftedness and a Church for all. These sections have raised the fundamental theological principles on which disability issues need to be viewed in the entire process of being Church.

The section on commonalities and differences underscores the need to consider the fact that people with disabilities are individuals with specific characteristics and not a homogeneous group that should just be seen in terms of provision of assistance and care. The hermeneutical issues section underscores the fact that disabilities need not just be viewed either as loss or as results of punishment for sin. They should be viewed as part of the human diversity and plurality of God's creation.

One over-riding theme in the Statement is that of the creation story as reflected by the section on Imago Dei. The section underscores the fact that it is not our intellect or our physical being which reflect the image of God in us. If this were the case, it would contradict the bible when it says "we are all created in the image of God." We are in a fragile world in which we are all part of the whole that reflects God's image. When God created the entire world, he saw that it was good. Thus, the notion that God's image has to do with our intellect or physical being is therefore a negation of his purpose. Christ himself bore a broken body on the cross which was the result of our salvation. In whatever state of being, we are wonderfully made–made in the image of God.

The healing section differentiates between healing and cure where the gospel healing stories are seen not as merely restoration of the body but more of the individual's restoration in, and into, society. It is an act of making them human and therefore joining up with the rest of the community in their day to day pre-occupation. When we create an inviting environment and provide space for full participation and active involvement of people with disabilities in the church life, we are participating in Christ's healing ministry.

The giftedness section highlights the fact that all of us, those with and without disabilities, are part of one Church and each has gifts and talent to contribute to being Church–gifts and talents without which the Church of Christ is not complete. The section on a Church for all (which is the last in the statement) highlights the necessity to accommodate the needs of all in worship, social, development, and political life of the Church. In worship, the statement maintains that it will be necessary to consider the needs of different categories of disabilities including good lighting, acoustics, sitting arrangement, sign language interpretation, and access not only to the building but also to the sanctuary. This is what a Church for all should be. One that accommodates everyone, accepts the gifts and talents that everyone brings and welcomes all irrespective of the differences that may threaten to set us aside from each other.

It is hoped that the text will demystify some of the disability discourse and will motivate more imaginative thinking about creating communities that encourage and facilitate the full participation of all people, including individuals with disabilities, in the spiritual and social life of the Church.

This document was received and adopted by the WCC Central Committee in August 2003 after a careful study and discussion by both the Central Committee itself and the Policy Reference Committee II. The document has been commended to all the member churches for study, feedback, and planning.

It is not possible to fathom the various reactions to some of these fundamental theological themes on which there might be different interpretations. The purpose of the Statement is not to impose any single interpretation to any or all of these themes but rather to encourage a discourse that will lead to better understanding of persons with disabilities, their needs and aspirations to facilitate their full participation and active involvement in the life of the Church.

CONCLUSION

As I have pointed in this document, religious faiths have been responsible for impressing on the idea of a merciful God who demands that human beings exercise this same virtue. In line with this idea, the Christian churches in the past have, especially in parts of the developing countries, established care centers which developed into educational and rehabilitation institutions. These were left in the hands of carers who maintained them in isolation with whatever else happened in the society. Those in such institutions remained closed up and therefore strangers to the rest of the society. This background has partly been responsible for a situation where social integration is not part of what the society understands.

As the Interim Statement notes, it is a fact that despite many years of addressing disability, the church has remained in a world where we have set up walls–walls that shut people in or shut people out, walls that prevent people from meeting and talking to others, and walls that keep many people from participating fully in life. Many people with disabilities still find themselves isolated behind walls of shame and fear, walls of ignorance and prejudice, walls of anger, walls of rigid dogma and cultural misunderstanding. This sad situation contradicts the fact that the Church is called to be one body. It is a fact that the churches are largely not conscious of these walls, which nevertheless negates the call to be one body through full participation.

The Disability Advocacy
of the National Council of Churches

Albert A. Herzog, Jr., PhD, MDiv, MA

SUMMARY. Since 1950, the National Council of Churches has worked ecumenically to foster numerous ministries among people with disabilities, both nationally and among its member communions. Its original emphasis was focused on the Christian education of children and adults with physical and developmental disabilities. Gradually, through exposure to other issues faced by persons with disabilities, and through involvement with secular and religious agencies, the Council's work expanded to include a wide variety of disability-related issues, including the International Year of Disabled Persons. Today, the Council's work involves denominational representatives beyond its member communions and has become increasingly integrated into the full agenda of the National Council of Churches. *[Article copies available for a fee from The Haworth Document Delivery Service: 1-800-HAWORTH. E-mail address: <docdelivery@haworthpress.com> Website: <http://www.HaworthPress.com> © 2006 by The Haworth Press, Inc. All rights reserved.]*

KEYWORDS. National Council of Churches, disability advocacy, Christian education of people with disabilities, International Year of Disabled Persons, ecumenism

---

Albert A. Herzog, Jr. is a Lecturer in Sociology at the Ohio State University, Newark, as well as an ordained minister in the United Methodist Church.

This article was based on research performed for the Committee on Disabilities of the National Council of Churches with financial support from the Religious Research Association.

[Haworth co-indexing entry note]: "The Disability Advocacy of the National Council of Churches." Herzog, Albert A. Jr. Co-published simultaneously in *Journal of Religion, Disability & Health* (The Haworth Pastoral Press, an imprint of The Haworth Press, Inc.) Vol. 10, No. 1/2, 2006, pp. 11-38; and: *Disability Advocacy Among Religious Organizations: Histories and Reflections* (ed: Albert A. Herzog, Jr.) The Haworth Pastoral Press, an imprint of The Haworth Press, Inc., 2006, pp. 11-38. Single or multiple copies of this article are available for a fee from The Haworth Document Delivery Service [1-800-HAWORTH, 9:00 a.m. - 5:00 p.m. (EST). E-mail address: docdelivery@haworthpress.com].

The National Council of the Churches of Christ in the USA (NCC) was established in 1950 by representatives of 29 Protestant and Orthodox denominations. Its organization was the result of a merger of twelve interdenominational agencies including the Federal Council of the Churches in America, the Home Missions Council of North America, and the International Council of Religious Education.[1]

The first preamble of the NCC constitution stated that the general or overall purpose of the Council was "to manifest oneness in Jesus Christ as Divine Lord and Savior, by the creation of an inclusive cooperative agency of the Christian Churches in the United States of America. . . . " The programs of the NCC were carried out by its divisions that were organized internally by departments, committees, and/or commissions. The Division of Christian Education was also organized in 1950 and assumed activities formerly undertaken by the International Council of Religious Education, the National Protestant Council on Higher Education, and the Missionary Education Movement of the United States and Canada. The inclusion of these organizations extended the work of the Division back as far as 1897.

THE NCC GETS STARTED

It is difficult to determine precisely when the Division of Christian Education began to consider disability issues. In 1954, it published "The Church and the Handicapped," a compilation of articles that had appeared in the *International Journal of Religious Education* over previous years. The booklet was introduced by Virgil E. Foster, who outlined the concerns addressed in the reprinted articles. After noting that "handicapped persons need spiritual and social nurture as much as the non-handicapped," Dr. Foster maintained that churches had been unaware of their responsibility to make such provisions as building access and assistive hearing devices as well as the "tragic lack of understanding of the *person* behind the handicap, and his need for what the church has to give." In addition, he outlined the three roles for the church in "unhandicapping the handicapped:"

> First of all, many handicaps are preventable. Churches need to be on the job in encouraging care in the prevention of accidents and exposure to crippling diseases. Many persons are not born with handicaps, but acquire them. The best way to unhandicap a person is to help him keep from becoming handicapped.

In the second place, many handicaps are wholly or partially curable. Cure is not achieved in many instances because of misunderstanding or lack of care. Conditions corrected in hospitals often appear again because of failure to maintain adequate discipline. The church, which is closer to many parents than any other influence, should be faithful and wise in its counsel in this matter.

In the third place, the biggest handicap faced by many persons is not the impairment but the spiritual and social starvation imposed by the community. The unhandicapping of the handicapped is a responsibility of churches. Central in the Christian message is the insistence upon the worth of every person in the sight of God and therefore in the sight of his fellows. Churches can help relieve many handicapped children, young people, and adults of this extra handicap. They can help them live fully in the areas of their normalcy, and increasingly in their areas of handicap.[2]

However, the Division's work with the Christian education of exceptional persons began in earnest in 1957 when a consultation was held on "the Churches' Responsibility for the Christian Education of Exceptional Persons" in Green Lake, Wisconsin. The report on this event provides both the background and the purpose for the gathering of 57 persons:[3]

Because of the growing interest and frequent requests for information the program committees of the Commission on General Christian Education of the National Council of Churches concurred in the request that a consultation be held to:

1. To arouse the churches to their responsibility for the Christian education of exceptional persons in the local church or in institutions.
2. In so far as possible to indicate some ways in which this responsibility may be fulfilled denominationally and/or inter-denominationally.

The consultation began with a "symposium" of "agency specialists" who spoke on "the Responsibility of the Church for the Christian Education of Exceptional Persons." Included on the list of speakers were representatives from several agencies including: the U.S. Department of Health, Education and Welfare; the National Society for Crippled Children and Adults; the American Foundation for the Blind;

the National Association for Retarded Children; the Council for Clinical Training; and the Office of County Superintendent of Schools, Waukesha, Wisconsin. A second preliminary session was devoted to presentations of six persons who described examples of what the church is "now doing for the Christian education of exceptional persons."[4]

The members of the consultation then divided into three "work groups" based on preferences indicated in advance: the physically handicapped; the mentally retarded; and "those under detention." Each group generated ideas and recommendations based on their internal discussions.

The work group on the physically handicapped recognized the need for education with respect to issues of disability at all levels of the church through sermons, print media, audio-visuals, and various hands-on projects. It recognized the dynamic nature of the population in that there were persons with physical handicaps in all age groups and life circumstances and that no two persons were alike in terms of response to their disabilities and needs. Also considered was the need to evaluate each individual so that only those who needed special programs would be separated from non-handicapped persons. The report from this group emphasized the need to deal with issues of rejection and acceptance within the context of the theological resources of the churches as well as the need to train the entire church with respect to the issues raised by the presence of people with physical handicaps and not only those who are directly involved in their care. Implications for all these concerns were listed according to possible efforts to be mounted at the national, state, community, and local church levels.

The work group on the "socially maladjusted and immature" focused on the need for the church to restudy its focus, especially with regard to "young people and adults of actual problem situations." Specifically, it raised five "action research" statements and questions:

1. What are the affects of the physical setting of the church on what has to be done with and for these maladjusted–recognizing that physical setup reveals our set of values?
2. Observe and record how the schedule, structure, kind of teaching affects the maladjusted–recognizing the need for flexibility with these people.
3. Observe and record the attitudes, ideas, and behavior of adults in the local church and discover how these affect the maladjusted.

4. What do Chaplains find are the needs in building relationships with children within an institution?
5. Influence public opinion, and legislation, work for adequate financial support, and program.

In addition, the work group presented a list of items entitled "what we would like to see happen" which included a "consultant psychological service for church school teachers and other church leaders," the development of Christian education materials for chaplains, the use of community resources and services, and the need to incorporate the previously institutionalized into the life of the local church.

The report from the work group on the mentally retarded began by outlining the current structure of work with the mentally retarded and their families as available in most communities. The work group focused on the role of the local association for retarded children which often established various task groups centering on community activities including religious life. A "sub-committee on orientation for the local church" listed "ways of making churches aware that there are such people in their congregations or communities, of developing (an) attitude that something can and should be done for them, of deciding what should be done and how to do it, and finally the resources available."

Another sub-committee focused on "ministering to the family with the child or adult who is retarded." In beginning its work, it listed some general assumptions upon which contact between the church and parents should be made:

1. Many parents have previously been hurt and have become suspicious before receiving help from the church.
2. This problem of parents may never be fully resolved and they may need support, encouragement and help over a long period of time.
3. More parents than the immediate family may be directly involved (i.e., grandparents, etc.).
4. Many times there has been inadequate professional counseling.

The sub-committee then outlined the essential features of the "church's contact with parents" including clergy and professional staff, the "church school teacher of the retarded child," the nursery home visitor, lay visitors, adult groups, and community organizations. It gave the church full responsibility in maintaining contact with the community in that "the church should do its full share in keeping the lines of communication open between itself and parent inspired groups so that these groups may know of the concern of the church and in turn the church may keep informed of needs and services."

Finally, the work group on mental retardation made a series of recommendations related to the "church school program for the child and adult," which were to have an impact on the future activities of the National Council of Churches. The first recommendation was "that age-level program committees, primarily CCW (Committee on Children's Work), initiate a study that would include research and experimentation looking toward guidance material for the Christian education of retarded persons." The work group then listed four areas that would be considered in this effort: "(1) exploration of religious needs and development of goals; (2) organization into groups, classes and other programs; (3) curriculum guidance and development; and (4) ways of working." This was followed be a series of detailed suggestions for each consideration. Interestingly, they indicated that, in a community where there were more than three children, a special class should be provided for the mentally retarded and not put in classes with normal children. In addition, they suggested that such a class "would best be done by an inter-church organization or by the local Association for Retarded Children on an inter-denominational basis."

In 1958, and in follow-up to the to the Green Lake, Wisconsin consultation, a Commission on Christian Education of Exceptional Persons was authorized, including a committee on the mentally retarded. This was chaired for many years by the Reverend Charles Palmer who was the Director of the Woodhaven Learning Center in Columbia, Missouri.[5] A basic "leadership text" *The Church and the Exceptional Person* was developed "to guide church leaders in understanding the characteristics and special needs of exceptional persons, and ways of involving them in religious programs."[6] The Commission also included working groups on "persons under custody of the law," physical handicaps, and persons with emotional disturbances.[7]

In 1960, the committee on mental retardation conducted a survey of religious programs through denominations, residential centers and regional state and local councils of churches. This led to the publication (in cooperation with Friendship Press) of a study titled *The Church's Mission and Persons of Special Need*. Additional information was gathered for special educators in 1961 and 1962 which led to the preparation of the manual Christian Education for Retarded Children and Youth published by Abingdon Press in 1963.[8]

Much of this work was accomplished through the Cooperative Publication Association (CPA), which involved representatives from the publishing organizations of 14 cooperating denominations. At the height of its operation in the 1950s, 60s and early 70s, the CPA acted as sounding board, clearing house, and facilitator for various publications having to do with persons with special needs (usually through a committee on mental retardation). These representatives would meet annually to discuss needs. Once the need for a particular piece was identified, one of the representatives would solicit the writing of the piece and oversee all matters pertaining to the publication's preparation. Upon completion, the article would be made available for use by publications of member denominations.

Using both frameworks (the Committees of the NCC and the Cooperative Publication Association) resulted in a series of very productive efforts on behalf of people with disabilities, and especially for people with mental retardation. In 1965, *The International Journal of Religious Education* published a special issue, "No Two Alike," which was designed to serve as a resource for leaders working with "special needs, including the retarded."[9] From 1965 through 1969, efforts were focused on the development of two curriculum series: "Adventures" and "Exploring Life." These were published through the Cooperative Publication Association on a national level with fourteen state councils of churches sponsoring introductory workshops to facilitate their use.

From 1969 through 1973, the work of the NCC with disabilities expanded to include other areas. A manual "Camping and the Mentally Retarded" was developed as an outgrowth of a consultation sponsored by the United Methodist Church. This resource shared insights by leaders experienced in programming with persons who were retarded in an outdoor setting as guidelines for developing new programs. Exploratory sessions were held with the American Bible Society on making the Scriptures "more useful" for persons with retardation which resulted in the publication of "Special Education Selections" and "Favorite Bible Selections." Other activities during this period included: (1) conversations with leaders in Black denominations to discuss special education opportunities and needs; (2) data gathering and sharing about church membership/confirmation practices for people with disabilities resulting in the preparation of an article "We Visited Leon Today" for use in church periodicals; (3) the development of "New Directions for Parents of Persons Who Are Retarded"; (4) mobilizing review panels to preview and evaluate audio-visuals to be incorporated in an audio-visual resource guide; (5) the gathering of success stories in a booklet "Let's Do More With Persons With Disabilities"; and (6) the development of an evaluation project to gather feedback from local users of the Adventure Series.[10] The committee continued conversations with leaders of agencies that served people with retardation including the National Association for Retarded Children and the American Association on Mental Deficiency (AAMD). In 1968, six committee members became members of the AAMD and its Subsection on Religion. Ima Jean Kidd (who had joined the NCC staff in 1959) was invited to present a paper on the NCC Department of Education's "Approach to the Religious Nurture of the Mentally Retarded."

The section of the "deaf and the gifted" indicated that descriptions for the task forces on "Christian education and the deaf" and "Christian education and the gifted" were prepared and presented to the Department of Education of the NCC. After a November, 1968 Executive Committee meeting, it was agreed to explore ways of staffing each task force with the possibility of "finding denominational staff persons who would undertake responsibilities for developing and administering task forces."

From 1974 through 1976, the NCC worked on filling the "gaps" based on the results of an evaluation project implemented through the Education Research staff of the Lutheran Church in America. This resulted in a number of projects including the development of six Supplemental Booklets for the "Adventure Series" published in 1976 through the Cooperative Publication Association. In addition, manuscripts were solicited for a new series of adult resources entitled the "Expanding World Series." The Committee also prepared a statement of philosophy and incorporated it into an article "They Have a Right to Live Among Us in Dignity."[11]

During these years the NCC worked in close cooperation with the Lutheran Church in America to develop a multi-media kit "Planning a Ministry with Persons Who Are Retarded" for use by congregations in designing and establishing local ministries. Also undertaken were consultations with national denominational staff who carried portfolios in human sexuality and/or family ministries in order to raise the need for a better understanding of human sexuality and the retarded. A working paper was produced entitled "The Rights of the Mentally Retarded in our Churches and Communities" and plans emerged for a series of workshops on "Human Sexuality and the Retarded" to be "church-sponsored in cooperation with universities and seminaries."

At the end of their presentation before the Religion Subdivision of the American Association of Mental Deficiency on May 30, 1976, the Reverend Charles Palmer and Ima Jean Kidd listed six areas which they felt needed consideration:

1. We have not yet come to grips with programs for the multiply handicapped. For a long time we have been discussing ways by which we could provide effective helps for parents of sons and daughters who are homebound, but have yet to come up with a suggested program.
2. We want to encourage churches to become more actively involved in day care and activity programs.
3. We have been concerned about the dismissal of adults from state residential facilities and their placement in nursing and group homes. We would like to devise some system to encourage the church to integrate their new community residents into the caring community of the church.
4. We are concerned about providing adequate parental supports. We think that such helps might be given through the pastor and the doctor, who are the first to know about the new-born retarded child. Assistance in development of counseling skills could come through seminary training and medical school studies.
5. We have concerns about mainstreaming. Too often all retarded are lumped together programmatically. We feel careful consideration should be given to the needs of each individual.
6. We have concerns for the education of the various publics. Generally speaking, most people are not aware of the many problems faced by retarded persons and their need to be helped to overcome them. Confusion still exists in the minds of many regarding mental illness and mental retardation. The Church has not fully realized its responsibility of ministering with all people, no matter how handicapped they are. Perhaps it is at this point that we all must work a little harder.

The authors closed their presentation with a comment that "we are sure you can think of many areas where the Church should be involved. We invite your comments." This, in effect, continued the NCC's reliance on the secular community of workers with the mentally retarded and the "exceptional person" for input and guidance. As they reflected on concerns about the impact of deinstitutionalization and community supports, they challenged the churches to respond to the needs of persons with various disabilities living in the community rather than dismissing them.

WORLD ECUMENISM

As the National Council of Churches moved toward the end of the 1970s, an additional focus was added to its work with disability-related issues. This had to do with the World Council of Churches and the United Nations declaration of 1981 as "The International Year for the Disabled (IYDP)."

As early as the presentation to AAMD, in 1976, the Reverend Charles Palmer and Ima Jean Kidd "rejoiced" in the report of the Fifth Assembly of the World Council of Churches, in Nairobi, Kenya in 1975, "What Unity Requires." The report adopted by the Assembly included a section entitled "The Handicapped and the Wholeness of the Family of God"[12] which affirmed the concepts of "equality and mutuality, human worth and personal dignity" with specific reference to persons with disabilities:

> The church cannot exemplify "the full humanity revealed in Christ," bear witness to the interdependence of humankind, or achieve unity in diversity if it continues to acquiesce in the social isolation of disabled persons and to deny them full participation in its life. The unity of the family of God is handicapped where these brothers and sisters are treated as objects of condescending charity. It is broken where they are left out.

All these efforts were highlighted when on November 9, 1977, the Governing Board of National Council of Churches adopted the "Resolution on the Church and Persons with Handicaps":[13]

> *Whereas* there are an estimated 35 million disabled Americans (7.8 million are children, at least 28 million adults with physical and mental handicaps*), and the first White House Conference on Handicapped Individuals was called and held in May 1977 to generate national awareness of problems facing handicapped citizens and to recommend policies and programs, and recent public laws have given major support to handicapped individuals (the 1973 Rehabilitation Act Public Law 93-112 and 1975 Public Law 94-142: Education for All Handicapped Children); and

> *Whereas* the United Nations General Assembly has adopted a Resolution (in December 1976) proclaiming the year 1981 as the "International Year for Disabled Persons"; and

> *Whereas* the World Council of Churches, in its Nairobi Assembly in late, 1975 adopted a report on "What Unity Requires" including a section on "The Handicapped and the Wholeness of the Family

of God," and asked the member churches to participate fully in a proposed WCC Study of the Church and the Disabled, and recommend that the churches "do everything possible to integrate the disabled into the life of the Church at every level"; and

Whereas several of the member communions of the National Council of Churches have taken actions at national assemblies in recent years lifting up the churches' responsibility in relation to persons with handicaps (i.e., United Methodist Church; Lutheran Church in America; United Presbyterian Church in the USA; and United Church of Christ); and

Whereas the year 1977 marks the twentieth anniversary of the first consultation called by the former Commission on General Christian Education (Division on Education and Ministry), and the Program Committee on Education for Christian Life and Mission (Division of Education and Ministry) has authorized a second consultation on "Church Education and Persons with Disabilities" for early 1978 to project future directions in educational ministry;

Therefore, the Governing Board of the National Council of the Churches of Christ in the U.S.A. applauds the progress and rejoices in the evidences of hope which are witnessed in the above international and national developments in church and society and reaffirms its belief in the dignity and worth of all persons, including persons with handicaps.

In addition, the Governing Board calls upon the member communions to increase efforts at all levels of church life (national, regional, local) toward full participation by persons with handicaps, through such means as providing appropriate educational programs, making necessary architectural modifications, being sensitive in the building of new structures to the needs of handicapped persons, overcoming attitudinal barriers, and developing advocacy programs in the church and society; and toward an end to discrimination against those with handicaps as well as those perceived by others as being physically and mentally handicapped.

*"Handicapped" is defined by the U.S. Department of Health, Education and Welfare to mean: "mentally retarded, hard of hearing, deaf, speech impaired, visually handicapped, seriously emotionally disturbed, crippled, or other health impaired persons."

This "Pronouncement" is significant for the history of the National Council of Churches work with disability issues in several important ways. First, it is the first resolution coming from the main governing body of the Council which focuses specifically on issues pertaining to disability. It is based on the "Pronouncement on Human Rights" which was adopted by the General Assembly on December 6, 1963.[14] This document provides a broad theological and social rationale for the church's concern for human rights and is tied to the "Universal Declaration of Human Rights" which was adopted without dissent in December, 1948 by the General Assembly of the United Nations.

The "Pronouncement on the Church and Persons with Handicaps" displays a heavy reliance on secular ideas and concepts about disability in use during the late 1970s. This is reflected, especially, in the use of terminology which served as the legal definition of "handicapped" as employed by the (then) U.S. Department of Health, Education and Welfare. However, the use of terms such as "handicapped," "mentally retarded," as well as other designations would change in the early 1980s. Perhaps more significant are its references to recently enacted federal laws pertaining to education of persons with a variety of handicapping conditions. The recognition and support of these measures plus change in focus would gradually move the NCC's work with disabilities toward the more general direction of disability rights.

On January 29 and 30th, 1980, a "Consultation on the International Year of Disabled Persons" was held at the Interchurch Center in New York City.[15] There were two stated goals of the Consultation. The first was "to provide a time for sharing projected plans for observing the IYDP including: the United Nations; the U.S. Council for IYDP; denominational groups; ecumenical groups." The second was to "identify two or three specific goals or projects that might be undertaken ecumenically and could make maximum impact; and to plan strategies for implementation." The list of invitations to this meeting was extensive including all the mainline Protestant denominations, several Orthodox communions, the Roman Catholic Church, ecumenical, and interested secular agencies.

The first part of the meeting was devoted to a review of information provided by the United Nations. The International Year for Disabled Persons as adopted by the United Nations General Assembly in 1975 sought to build upon previous efforts, reaffirming its "deep-rooted faith in human rights and fundamental freedoms, principles of peace, the dignity and worth of the human person, and the promotion of social justice, as proclaimed by the Charter of the United Nations." In addition, the

U.N. recalled three previous declarations regarding persons with disabilities: (1) a resolution from December, 1971 "proclaiming the Declaration on the Rights of Mentally Retarded Persons"; (2) a resolution from December, 1975 "proclaiming the Declaration on the Rights of Disabled Persons"; and (3) a resolution of December, 1976 "on the implementation of the Declaration on the Rights of Disabled Persons."[16]

Each denominational representative reported on their activities with regard to IYDP usually in the context of their ongoing ministries with persons with various disabilities. The meeting also included participation and reports from several ecumenical groups including: Church Women United; the John Milton Society for the Blind; Mainstream: In Church and Society; the Healing Community; the World Council of Churches; as well as the National Council of Churches. Of these, The Healing Community was perhaps the most innovative. It introduced its packet "The Caring Congregation" (which was also the theme of new book by its Director, the Reverend Dr. Harold Wilke, enititled "Creating the Caring Congregation") as well as its work on Access Sunday. In addition, Dr. Wilke emphasized the meeting and activities of Rehabilitation International and the development of Chapter VII–"Inclusive Ministry," a paper for the Consultation on Church Union.

The Consultation set the goal "Toward Full Participation of all Disabled Persons in Church and Society" with the projects in three areas: (1) finding jobs for disabled persons, who are presently unemployed; (2) providing for adequate transportation in each community; and (3) lifting up education opportunities. At the conclusion of the Consultation, the Education for Christian Life and Mission Program Committee of the National Council of Churches agreed to coordinate and communicate the development of resources for the IYDP. Its newsletter *Embracing Diversity* would be published more often in 1980 and 1981. In addition, "update memos" would carry information about resources and models.

On November 8, 1980, the Governing Board of the National Council of Churches adopted a "Resolution on International Year of Disabled Persons" (1981). As in its previous resolution on persons disabilities, the statement summarized the work of the NCC:

> *Whereas* the United Nations has proclaimed 1981 as the International Year of Disabled Persons and has invited all nations to establish concrete goals and programs aimed at improving the quality of life for persons with disabilities; and

Whereas President Carter has commended the initiative of the private sector in planning the U.S. program for the 1981 Year observance and has pledged both his personal support and that of the Administration for the U.S. effort; and

Whereas a U.S. Council has been formed to promote, through community commitment, full participation by persons with disabilities in all aspects of society, has established long-term goals not only to increase public awareness of the unmet needs of persons with disabilities but also to improve the quality of their lives, and in support of the work of the Year, has adopted the slogan "Meeting the Challenges Through Partnerships"; and

Whereas the formulation of action-oriented programs and the development of partnerships within the community between persons with and without disabilities, state and local governments, and local organizations should be the outgrowth of community commitment and should facilitate the integration of persons with disabilities into society; and

Whereas the National Council of Churches adopted a "Resolution on the Church and Persons with Handicaps" on November 9, 1977, calling on member communions to increase efforts at all levels of church life (national, regional, local) toward full participation by persons with handicaps . . . ; and

Whereas the National Council of Churches and several of the member communions have already joined the U.S. Council for the International Year of Disabled Persons as national partners; and

Whereas the Program Committee, Education for Christian Life and Mission (Division of Education and Ministry), held a Consultation on January 29-30, 1980 to consider ways churches might observe the International Year of Disabled Persons, and has developed guidelines for local congregations and challenges our churches to use the 1981 observance as a springboard for increasing efforts toward "full participation of all disabled persons in church and society";

Therefore be it resolved that the Governing Board of the National Council of Churches of Christ in the U.S.A.:

1. *Supports* the worldwide objective of the United Nations to establish goals and programs that will enrich the lives of citizens with disabilities; and
2. *Supports* the aims of the U.S. Council to fully integrate such people into community life, to target the limited financial resources of our churches and country to the most productive uses and to sharpen public awareness of the problems and needs of persons with disabilities.

The impact of the IYDP is easy to see for a least two reasons. First, as early as the fall of 1980 inquires began coming into the Special Learning Needs Office requesting resources for National Family Week in 1981. In response, the NCC, several denominational groups, and other interest groups developed the theme "Families of Special Need" as a focus for the following year as a part of the observance of the IYDP. Second, the work of the NCC became closely tied to such organizations as the National Organization on Disability and other ecumenical agencies such as the World Council of Churches.[17] This was especially with regard to the establishment of the Decade of Persons with Disabilities (1983-1992) which continued the program of action set up by the 1981 IYDP. In this, the NCC endorsed The Healing Community's development of "A Call to Action within The Decade of Persons with Disabilities (1983-1992), for Church, Synagogue, Temple, and Mosque." The Healing Community's goals for the Decade became important as it developed and distributed resources used by ecumenical groups (including the NCC), denominations, and congregations:

1. Access, physical and attitudinal, to and within church, synagogue, temple, and mosque, with adequate transportation for religious and secular purposes.
2. Expanded religious education at all age levels, and community education leading toward better understanding of the impact of disability, congenital and acquired, seen and unseen.
3. Expanded employment opportunity within religious groups, and in the secular community with help from lay leaders of the congregation in business and industry.
4. Expanded participation in recreational, social, religious and cultural activities, both within the religious group and beyond.
5. Expanded and international use of the concept of "the congregation as a healing community," thereby enhancing the work of rehabilitation programs and facilities.

6. Application of research in substance abuse, environmental impact, accident prevention and other areas, all aimed at reducing or even eliminating major disabling conditions.
7. Reductions of disability through clearer affirmation of a positive lifestyle which supports family life and affirms the values of religious life.
8. Advocacy for young, aging, and disabled persons in community living programs and other aspects of community life.
9. Expanded international exchange of information and experience to benefit disabled persons of all faiths.[18]

THE WORK CONTINUES

During the 1980s, the NCC Task Force on Mental Retardation (which, at its February, 1984 annual work session) voted to change its name to Task Force on Developmental Disabilities in order "to broaden the scope of (its) responsibilities") met at various locations in the United States while the Mental Retardation/Developmental Disability Committee of the Cooperative Publication Association usually met in late Fall. Both the minutes of the Task Force and Cooperative Publication Association indicate an on-going pattern which had been established in prior decades. There was an honest attempt to grapple with serious issues impacting on the disability community. In addition to the concern for deinstitutionalization, other issues such as mainstreaming, citizen advocacy, and human sexuality for persons with mental retardation (gradually moving to the use of the term "persons with developmental disabilities") emerged for consideration.[19]

As previously, the NCC sought to come to terms with these developments by receiving direct input from secular experts. For instance, in the late 1980s, the Task Force considered the issue of mental retardation and human sexuality. Consultants were brought in from The Coalition on Sexuality and Disability, Inc. to discuss current research, policy and programs provided by secular agencies. These consultants attended meetings of the Task Force for several years and offered additional insights including critiques of denominational statements on mental retardation and human sexuality. In response, the Task Force discussed the implications of these inputs for its work as well as the work of the denominations. On many occasions, issues discussed at the Task Force meeting in the Spring would become part of the agenda of the CPA meeting the following Fall as new resources were contemplated.

In addition to the Task Force on Developmental Disabilities proper, there were also "work groups" established to deal with specific issues. In February, 1984, it established a work group on autism to "gather information, analyze learnings and consider needs for strategies and guidance for church leaders." The February, 1985 meeting of the work group (to be held in conjunction with the annual meeting of the Task Force on Developmental Disabilities) would be devoted to the tasks of "updating about modern trends; reviewing definitions of autism; looking at characteristics; and gathering case studies about programs sponsored by religious groups."[20]

In Fall, 1987 *Embracing Diversity* reported on a "Consultation on Language, Thought and Social Justice and Persons with Disabilities"[21] which "took a long look at the links joining language, thought and social justice." Two scheduled workshops focused, particularly, on persons with disabilities. The first, "Disabled . . . Handicapped . . . and in the Image of God?" explored "how language affects our theology, faith development and spirituality in marginalizing people with disabilities." The second, "Language Insights from the Deaf Communication Styles" focused on "various communication modes of deaf persons (which) influence their thinking and their culture." On the workshops, Dr. Arthur O. Van Eck, the NCC's Associate General Secretary for Education and Ministry, commented: "this consultation grew out of continuing work that the Division of Education and Ministry had done toward a more inclusive church. A major focus of our efforts has been to create resources for worship and education that use language inclusive of men and women, of ethnic minority persons, of all ages and of persons with disabilities."[22]

As the result of the Consultation, the Fall, 1988 edition of *Embracing Diversity* focused on the theme "cultural diversity and persons with disabilities." Topics covered in the newsletter included (among others): a discussion of the Ethnic Minority Concerns Committee of the National Alliance for the Mentally Ill (NAMI); a brief article on Chinese-American families with children with disabilities; a discussion of resources on multi-culturalism available through the Council for Exceptional Children; and an article about Native Americans who use wheelchairs.[23]

Another milestone during this period was the NCC's involvement in the creation of Pathways to Promise: Interfaith Ministries and Prolonged Mental Illness. This organization emerged as an outgrowth of a "Consultation on the Church's Ministry with Persons who are Chronically Mentally Ill and their Families" held in St. Louis, June 25-27, 1987. The Consultation gathered seventy-seven denominational staff members, local clergy, family members, and consumers of mental health services. Its major finding was that "faith communities are key in the ongoing health of persons who have long-term mental illnesses, and who are striving to live full and meaningful lives in the community." The gathering was made possible by a grant from The Lutheran Charities Foundation of sixty-one St. Louis congregations of the Lutheran Church-Missouri Synod.[24]

However, it was after a second consultation a year later in Boulder, Colorado, entitled Pathways to Promise, which resulted in the "formation of an interfaith coalition to aid religious communities in providing more profound religious care of and ministry with persons who are seriously mentally ill and their families." Again, this was made possible by the presence of Ima Jean Kidd representing the NCC and others to form a group whose main activities were to provide the theological and "enabling" resources necessary for congregations to respond to the seriously mentally ill. As the news release on the organization of Pathways to Promise indicated: "the emergence of an Interfaith Coalition at the Boulder conference now promotes a birthing of an increased marching forth by the interfaith community toward the promising horizon of greater hope and programming on behalf of the mentally ill."[25]

INTO THE LAST DECADE

The most dramatic event of the late 1980s and early 1990s was the retirement of Ima Jean Kidd, who, as director of Special Learning Needs, had joined the National Council of Churches staff in 1959. Building on the pioneer work of several staff members including Alice Goddard, Virgil Foster, Mary Venable, J. Blaine Fister, and Alcwyn L. Roberta, Ms. Kidd spearheaded the numerous activities and events as well as the development of many of the resources described previously. For the most part, indications of her personal leadership are to be found in her reports, minutes, and other descriptions of the events sponsored and/or initiated by the Division of Education and Ministry (later Education for Christian Life and Mission). On May 2, 1968, Ima Jean Kidd concluded a speech to the Subsection on Religion of the American Association of Mental Deficiency (now Mental Retardation) entitled "An Approach to Religious Nurture of the Mentally Retarded"[26] with the following observations:

> Partnership across professional lines not only strengthens the quality of a product, but provides opportunity for enriching personal ex-

periences. How often we admit that we spend too much time talking with each other, and then continue life in our "professional ghettos."

Doors can be opened through individual people and organizational channels if time is taken to search and knock. We have discovered a number of persons who are willing to invest large amounts of time, often with minimal reimbursement, in order for a program of this kind to become a reality.

We must continue our work in the mode of experimentation, evaluation and humility. We were reminded of that fact upon hearing from an administrator of a residential center, who had been asked to review descriptions for the educable series. He commented: "My overall impression of the materials is good, I think you are on the 'right track.' But remember, when all this is done, you have only just begun!"

In actuality, the transition to a new era began a year or so earlier when the Task Force on Developmental Disabilities listed its goals for 1988-1991,[27] the transition period:

1. To advocate for the active participation of persons with developmental disabilities in church and society; and to develop resources/strategies that will encourage that involvement.
2. To broaden the information base for ministry with persons with developmental disabilities through sharing and evaluating resources, program models, research studies, and denominational priorities and policies.
3. To enable denominational representatives to participate in joint projects, such as leadership programs, and media development.
4. To provide for in-service education during annual meetings.
5. To relate to other groups working in the area of disability concerns.
6. To extend invitations, and to involve additional denominations for representation on the task force.

Along with these was a list of strategies which further clarified the role of the Task Force:

1. To maintain the group's focus on "developmental disabilities" (DD), including mental retardation, epilepsy, cerebral palsy, and autism.

2. To continue explorations and sharing regarding human sexuality and persons with developmental disabilities.
3. To explore ways to provide input into NCC-ECLM 1991 "Families 2000" event.
4. To promote the education of seminarians and clergy regarding disability concerns.
5. To continue work on the advocacy/friendship program concept and model.
6. To continue explorations regarding medical care/genetic issues, and counseling possibilities.
7. To continue efforts to articulate theological issues.
8. To find ways to review/monitor pending legislation as it pertains to persons with developmental disabilities.
9. To produce and disseminate resources on mainstreaming and new curriculum materials.
10. To promote expansion of the concept of respite care and supportive care/guardianship within the churches, and to monitor progress and learnings.
11. To collect art and photographs done by persons with DD, or appropriate for use in illustrating persons with DD.
12. To investigate logistics and to consider developing strategies for displays and involvement at annual meetings of secular organizations working with DD.

These goals and strategies outline a comprehensive program of activities and action that were soon placed into the limitations of funding, staff availability, and NCC reorganization. By its 1991 Annual Meeting, the Task Force on Developmental Disabilities was placed in "Ministries in Christian Education," as a "project" under Special Learning Needs. Ms. Alonna Gautsche Sprunger had been hired on contract to staff the Task Force which, according to the 1988-1991 Task Force "job description," allowed for approximately 15 days of staff time a year.[28]

Nevertheless, the "heavy" agenda of the Task Force continued. The 1991 Annual Meeting was convened in Grand Rapids, Michigan[29] where Tom Hocksema presented "five areas in special education" where the church could have an impact: (1) inclusive education; (2) preparation for work; (3) providing educational advocates besides the parents for children with disabilities in regular or special classroom settings; (4) thinking of ways for Christian institutions of higher education to comply "to the same standards of inclusiveness as secular institutions of higher education"; and (5) "brainstorm on how to bring young people into professions in the field of disabilities." Presentations were also made by Marilyn Bishop of the Center for Ministries with Disabled People, University of Dayton on seminary and clergy education, Marlys Taege from the National Christian Resource Center on Mental Retardation (who provided an overview of its program), and Ginny Thornburgh from the National Organization on Disability. Mrs. Thornburgh provided an overview of the civil rights provisions of the Americans With Disabilities Act (ADA) and led a discussion of the implications of the apparent exemption of religious organizations and/or organizations operated by religious organizations. The Task Force concluded its meeting by setting "Quadrennial Goals . . . Beginning to Plan for the Next Four Years" which listed twelve "possible directions" in terms of programs and policy development:

1. Concentrate on the most vulnerable.
2. Church inclusion (relationships and friendships).
3. Demythologize.
4. Self-advocacy.
5. Inclusive–regular education in church and public schools.
6. Sexuality–supportive marriages and supported parenting.
7. ADA and the church.
8. Theological issues–need language to execute the gospel.
9. Seminary and clergy training.
10. Dilemma of reduction in federal and state funding.
11. "Abiding in Faith" curriculum: A Resource for Teachers of Adults with Moderate Mental Retardation.
12. Family issues (siblings, divorce rates of parents, respite care, etc.).

The 1992 and 1993 Task Force meetings focused on seminary education and the development of the "Abide in Faith" curriculum. Marilyn Bishop continued as a consultant for seminary education and Tom Hocksema as consultant for special education. At the 1993 Task Force meeting a discussion was held on its name. After a lengthy discussion, a decision was made to change the name Task Force on Developmental Disabilities to NCC Committee on Disabilities "with an understanding that our mission statement include a priority on developmental disabilities."[30]

The 1994 NCC Committee on Disabilities met in Dayton, Ohio where "Models for Denominational Disability Ministries in the 90s" was added as a third work group to seminary education and "Curriculum and Inclusive Christian Education." After the business meeting adjourned, a symposium was held on "Ministry Perspectives on Disability." In addition, and upon the resignation of Alonna Gautsche Sprunger, a search was launched for a new contract staff and Joe Leonard began service as the NCC staff liaison to the Committee. Marilyn Bishop was selected to be the new contract staff person.[31]

On October 9-11, 1995, Marilyn Bishop and Jim Vanderlaan (chair of the NCC Committee on Disabilities) attended a meeting of the National Ministries Unit of the NCC. Both spoke to the entire group to explain the work of the committee. They also distributed a six-page paper entitled "Burning Issues" which "demonstrated that all current issues addressed by various units of the NCC have a disability component." For each burning issue they provided "an explanatory statement, a corroborating statement from a denominational resolution on disabilities, a quote from a relevant journal plus a comment from a member of the committee on disabilities" in order to "show that the issue of disability pervades all other concerns in society." In conclusion, both participants indicated a need for the Committee to work more closely with the National Ministries Unit in an attempt to impact member committees on disability issues.[32]

At its meeting in March, 1995, the NCC Committee on Disabilities elected to seek funding to develop an NCC policy statement on inclusion of persons living with disabilities to be presented ultimately to the NCC General Governing Board for approval. This was prepared and ready for discussion at the Committee's 1996 meeting.[33] In essence, the policy statement updates past resolutions which sought to bring the NCC into the mainstream of secular as well as religious disability policy.

NCCC POLICY STATEMENT ON DISABILITIES, THE BODY OF CHRIST, AND THE WHOLENESS OF SOCIETY

"Indeed, the body does not consist of one member but of many."

(I Cor. 12:14)

One in five Americans lives with an impairment that significantly limits one or more major life activities. Virtually everyone will live with a disability at some time in life. Concepts of justice for people with disabilities have evolved beyond paternalism toward the ideals of full participation and inclusion in all aspects of life. Disability rights and self advocacy movements have emerged. At the national level, landmark laws such as the Rehabilitation Act, The Individuals with Disabilities Education Act (IDEA), and the Americans With Disabilities Act (ADA) seek to assure the same rights to people with disabilities that are guaranteed to all other people in our society.

The religious community has also taken a number of initiatives. Beginning in 1958 and as recently as 1990, the NCCC has affirmed its belief in the dignity and worth of all people, including those of us with disabilities. Most NCCC member communions have listed statements calling for the full inclusion of people with disabilities in all aspects of church life. In spite of these efforts, attitudinal, communications, and architectural barriers remain. The church has served as a point of entry for many marginalized individuals into the main stream of society. Now the time has come for the NCC to reaffirm and broaden its commitment to people with disabilities.

This policy statement rests upon four theological principles:

1. All people are created in the image of God

"So God created humankind in his image . . . " (Gen. 1:27)

God creates all human beings in the divine image or likeness. This image is not a measurable characteristic or set of characteristics. God's image is reflected differently in each person.

2. All people are called by God

"For we are what he has made us, created in Christ Jesus for good works, which God prepared beforehand to be our way of life." (Eph 2:10)

God calls all human beings to express the divine image through their unique characteristics. Each person's characteristics, including disabilities, are inseparable and valuable features of the unique, indivisible person.

3. **All people have special gifts**

"Now there are varieties of gifts but the same spirit . . . " (1 Cor. 12:4)

God supplies all human beings with the unique gifts needed to obey the divine call. The gifts God has given to each person are needed by all other people, and no one is dispensable or unnecessary.

4. **All people are invited to participate in God's ministry**

"To each is given the manifestation of the Spirit for the common good." (I Cor. 12:7)

God invites all human beings to rely on and participate in the ministry of the Church. God continually empowers each member of the Body of Christ to reflect the divine image in ways that will serve and benefit the Church and the broader community.

Implications

In the light of these theological principles, it is the witness of the NCCC that all human beings, including those among us with disabilities, are entitled by God to the rights implied in the divine call. These rights include a life of dignity and respect with access to education, health care, useful work, recreation, as well as the right to friendship, spiritual nurture, freedom, and self-expression. The rights of each person, including people with disabilities, are equal to and balanced by the rights of others.

We believe the human community in all its forms is accountable to God to protect these civil and human rights. God requires the church to give spiritual and moral leadership to society in protecting these rights. The church must exercise its leadership by its public preaching and teaching but even more by its example as an inclusive community of faith, using the gifts of all of its members.

"Now there are varieties of gifts but the same spirit; and varieties of services, but the same Lord . . . " (I Cor. 12:4)[34]

In April, 1997, the Committee met at Princeton Theological Seminary with "Thematic Conversations Regarding Disability within the Framework of Courses of Worship, Scripture, Pastoral Care" being the theme and focus of the event. This continued the Committee's work on seminary-related issues.[35] Later that year, the NCCC Policy Statement received its first reading before the Governing Board with a second reading scheduled for late the next year. In the interim and before its annual meeting, the executive committee of the Committee on Disabilities pondered whether "concrete implications of the policy statement should be spelled out." The executive committee decided that "implications ought not be part of the policy statement itself, but that specific resolutions ought to be developed on the basis provided by the policy statement." Subsequently, one of the members was engaged to write a document on "assisted suicide and the quality of life." As stated in a letter by Committee Chair James Vanderlaan, "the document will clearly express concern about the growing acceptance of assisted suicide to terminate the life of a person who is disabled whose quality of life is therefore deemed so low that suicide is considered an acceptable option. The document will articulate a moral stance against using any socially imposed quality of life standard as a reason to justify assisted suicide."[36]

At the 1999 annual meeting, the NCC Committee on Disabilities once again established long-term and short-term goals. The long-term goals were set for four years and are as follows:

- To increase the number of seminaries that have disability ministry issues addressed in courses.
- To encourage publication, distribution, and sharing of video and print resources.
- To use the internet to distribute information.
- To present workshops on spiritual access at secular conferences.
- To restructure the annual meeting format to increase full participation for the entire meeting.

The following one-year goals were then set at the next day's meeting:

1. To re-structure the annual meeting format so that all members stay for the entire meeting.
2. To pursue and support the initiative proposed by Bill Gaventa regarding theological education.
3. To ask individual members to report on their progress toward achieving the goals.

4. To adopt the Abilities Expo to do a workshop and a display at locations throughout the United States.[37]

At the 2000 annual meeting these and other issues were discussed. However, as those present enjoyed the beauty of Puget Sound, there was the recognition that the NCC Committee on Disabilities is truly ecumenical in that many of the regular participants are from communions outside the membership of the NCC. These participate because there is no other group that meets nationally and ecumenically. In addition to the contributions of all present (including consultants such as Ginny Thornburgh from the National Organization on Disability and Bill Gaventa from the Religion Division of the American Association of Mental Retardation), the Committee on Disabilities is providing more input into the larger bodies of Ministries in Christian Education and the NCC Governing Board. Such efforts are extremely important as the National Council of Churches of Christ seeks, at all levels, both to broaden the ecumenical table and to address such issues a poverty in America.

As the 2001 annual meeting of the NCC Committee on Disabilities approached (which was actually held in March 2002 because of the horrific events of September 11, 2001), many issues remained unsettled including Bill Gaventa's proposal "Enhancing Theological and Professional Education in Spiritual Supports for Persons with Disabilities" and the piece on "Assisted Suicide and Quality of Life with Disabilities."[38] These emphases were deemed essential for the future of the churches' response to people with disabilities. In preparation for these visits, the 2001 meeting in Atlanta heard Nancy Eieisland speak about current issues in the "theology of disability." At the 2003 meeting in Grand Rapids, members of the Committee lectured to the students at Calvin Seminary and presented papers at a faculty forum where approximately 100 students, faculty and people from the community had gathered.[39]

The 2004 meeting at Union Theological Seminary in New York City would again emphasize the importance of theological education as well as the role of the Committee in the larger work of the National Council of Churches. It would establish ties between it and the World Council of Churches, especially with respect to its "interim statement," *A Church of All and for All*, written by its Ecumenical Disability Advocate Network (EDAN). It would, among other initiatives, "lift up, commend, and publicize the document from the Massachusetts Council of Churches, *The Accessible Church: Toward Becoming the Whole Family of God, Opportunities and Responsibilities for Ministry with People with Disabilities,"* and pledge to "further seminary education specifically by working with the Henri Nouwen Society."[40]

As it looked ahead, plans were made to "participate in and plan a gathering for representatives from major religious networks and organizations that work in the area of ministries and support with people with disabilities at a national disability summit in Washington, D.C. September 20-24, 2005."[41] One is reminded of what was said by Ima Jean Kidd and Charles Palmer over twenty-five years ago: "we feel that our task is not finished, and perhaps it never will be."[42] Yet, the disability advocacy of the National Council of Churches has progressed from the agendas of Christian educators to involvement of persons with disabilities and their advocates, from a focus on nurture to a focus on rights and inclusion. The tasks are without end, but the concern and motivation is still alive.

NOTES

1. "Brief History of the National Council of Churches," NCC Finding Aid/Collection Guide, National Council of Churches Archives at the Presbyterian Historical Society, 1.

2. Virgil E. Foster, "Introduction: Unhandicapping the Handicapped." The Church and the Handicapped. New York: National Council of Churches, 1954.

3. The material from the Consultation was derived from an unpublished report entitled, "Consultation on the Churches' Responsibility for the Christian Education of Exceptional Persons," held at the American Baptist Assembly at Green Lake, Wisconsin, October 4-5, 1957.

4. See below.

5. Personal Communication, Ima Jean Kidd, May 22, 2002.

6. Palmer, Charles and Ima Jean Kidd. "Two Decades of Cooperative Efforts in Ministry with the Mentally Retarded." Paper presented to the opening session of the American Association of Mental Deficiency, May 30, 1976, Chicago, IL.

7. Kidd, Ima Jean. "Religious Education and Persons with Disabilities." (no date).

8. This information is contained in the Palmer/Kidd paper. (See note #6).

9. Note on this article needed here.

10. This information is contained in the Palmer/Kidd paper. (See note #6).

11. This information is contained in the Palmer/Kidd paper. (See note #6).

12. This reference was derived from Minutes of General Synod of the United Church of Christ, 1977.

13. Copied from separate sheet.

14. "Pronouncement on Human Rights." Adopted by the General Assembly, December 6, 1963.

15. This information is derived from "Minutes: Consultation on the UN International Year of Disabled Persons," January 29-30, 1980 in New York, NY.

16. This information is attached to the Minutes described in Note #20.

17. Kidd, Ima Jean, "Introduction" (single sheet dated January, 1981).

18. The Caring Congregation–Quarterly periodical of The Healing Community (Combined issue, Vol. V:4 and Vol 6:1 (no date).

19. These observations are taken from notes of the meetings by the author of this report.

20. Embracing Diversity (various issues).

21. Embracing Diversity, Vol. 9:3 (Fall, 1987).

22. "Consultation on Language, Thought and Social Justice and Persons with Disabilities," *Embracing Diversity*, Fall, 1987, Vol 3, No. 3, 2.

23. Embracing Diversity, Vol. 10:3 (Fall, 1988).

24. Report: Consultation on the Church's Ministry with Persons who are Chronically Mentally Ill and their Families, June 25-27, 1987.

25. Fowler, Ruth. "New Religious Coalition for the Mentally Ill Organized." (7/30/88).

26. Kidd, Ima Jean. "An Approach to Religious Nurture of the Mentally Retarded," paper presented to the Subsection on Religion of the American Association of Mental Deficiency, May 2, 1968.

27. Separate Memo (no date).

28. See Minutes of Task Force on Developmental Disabilities, 1991.

29. See Minutes of Task Force on Developmental Disabilities, 1992.

30. See Minutes of the NCC Committee on Disabilities, 1993.

31. See Minutes of the NCC Committee on Disabilities, 1994.

32. Bishop, Marilyn E. and James Vanderlaan, "Report and Reflection on National Ministries Consultation, Pawling, New York, October 9-11, 1995."

33. See Minutes of the NCC Committee on Disabilities, 1996.

34. Copied from Separate Sheet.

35. See Minutes of the NCC Committee on Disabilities, 1997.

36. Vanderlaan, James, "Letter to Members, NCC Committee on Disabilities, March 20, 1998.

37. See Minutes of the NCC Committee on Disabilities, 1999.

38. See Minutes of the NCC Committee on Disabilities, 2000.

39. Minutes of the NGC Committee on Disabilities, 2003.

40. 2004 Annual Report of the NCC Committee on Disabilities to the Education and Leadership Ministries Commission.

41. 2004 Annual Report of the NCC Committee on Disabilities to the Education and Leadership Ministries Commission.

42. Palmer, Charles and Ima Jean Kidd, "Two Decades of Cooperative Efforts in Ministry with the Mentally Retarded." (See Note #6).

The Evolution and Current Focus of Ministry with Catholics with Disabilities Within the United States

Michelle N. Baum, BA
Janice L. Benton, sfo, BA

SUMMARY. The authors provide an historical overview of outreach to Catholics with disabilities within the U.S., including the contributions of early pioneers in the ministry. They also describe the founding of the National Catholic Partnership on Disability and its current activities and future directions, as well as the work of numerous Catholic ministry partners. *[Article copies available for a fee from The Haworth Document Delivery Service: 1-800-HAWORTH. E-mail address: <docdelivery@haworthpress.com> Website: <http://www.HaworthPress.com> © 2006 by The Haworth Press, Inc. All rights reserved.]*

KEYWORDS. Disability, Catholic, ministry, religion and disability

---

Michelle N. Baum is a freelance writer and mother of three children based in Fairlee, VT.

Janice L. Benton, the Executive Director of the National Catholic Partnership on Disability, has been a disability advocate for nearly three decades.

[Haworth co-indexing entry note]: "The Evolution and Current Focus of Ministry with Catholics with Disabilities Within the United States." Baum, Michelle N., and Janice L. Benton. Co-published simultaneously in *Journal of Religion, Disability & Health* (The Haworth Pastoral Press, an imprint of The Haworth Press, Inc.) Vol. 10, No. 1/2, 2006, pp. 39-54; and: *Disability Advocacy Among Religious Organizations: Histories and Reflections* (ed: Albert A. Herzog, Jr.) The Haworth Pastoral Press, an imprint of The Haworth Press, Inc., 2006, pp. 39-54. Single or multiple copies of this article are available for a fee from The Haworth Document Delivery Service [1-800-HAWORTH, 9:00 a.m. - 5:00 p.m. (EST). E-mail address: docdelivery@haworthpress. com].

Available online at http://www.haworthpress.com/web/JRDH
© 2006 by The Haworth Press, Inc. All rights reserved.
doi:10.1300/J095v10n01_04

HISTORICAL OVERVIEW

When and where did the American Catholic response to disability begin? In 1978, when the U.S. Catholic Bishops issued a call for full inclusion of persons with disabilities in the life of the Church and community? Or in the late sixties during the push for deinstitutionalization when small residential homes were begun through Catholic Charities? In 1966, when Special Religious Education (SPRED) was established to design and implement religious education curricula for people with developmental disabilities or as Cardinal Stritch College in Milwaukee, WI began a Masters Degree program in Special Religious Education? Or in 1837, when two Sisters of St. Joseph of Carondelet came from Lyons, France, to join six Sisters who emigrated the previous year at the request of Bishop Joseph Rosati of St. Louis to open a school in his diocese and welcomed four deaf students to study with the hearing students?

In truth, the Catholic response to disability is a long, rich, and ongoing story, one that covers a journey from ignorance and fear, through compassion and charity, and on into an inclusiveness that recognizes not only the dignity of Catholics with assorted disabilities but the gifts and insight they offer. Disability ministry within the Church has grown to include not only ministries *to* Catholics with disabilities but *among*, *with*, and *from* them.

The most recent manifestation of inclusive ministry within the Catholic Church was in the creation of the National Catholic Office for Persons with Disabilities (NCPD) in 1982 (renamed the National Catholic Partnership on Disability in 2002), whose ongoing work serves to promote consciousness and provide resources for Catholics with disabilities and their families nationally. NCPD has, since its inception, worked to provide support to diocesan directors in their efforts to create access and opportunities within the Church for Catholics with disabilities.

However, before NCPD was established, and before the U.S. Bishops' 1978 *Pastoral Statement on People with Disabilities* that was its source, came scores of organizations and thousands of people whose pioneering work broke important ground for both the Church and society. Residential programs, schools and religious education programs were developed to serve the needs of children with disabilities, particularly those who were deaf or who had cognitive disabilities. The Church often led the way in recognizing the dignity of each person, regardless of their disability. As Grace Harding, former director of the Office for Persons with Disabilities in the Diocese of Pittsburgh explains: "Historically religious orders served as a place of sanctuary for people with cognitive disabilities. They took in people with little fanfare in recognition of the value of their life. I see that time as 'The Age of Protection,' while this current time I consider the 'Age of Proclamation' in which we are proclaiming the gifts people bring to their Church communities."

In the earliest history of the Church, and indeed in the world as a whole, persons with disabilities were often held with fear and scorn, in practice if not in doctrine. Running parallel with society, Catholic focus on the needs and dignity of people with disabilities was far from ideal. However, as the social consciousness of the nation rose, so did that of the Church. In fact, according to Sr. Bernadette Downes, former board member and Chair of NCPD and longtime advocate, the Church often led by example in the growing movement for the right of people with disabilities to not only basic human dignity but the right to participate in the decisions affecting their lives. This leadership came from both the grassroots level and Church hierarchy and was rooted in the basic Catholic teaching of love of neighbor and the recognition that every human being is created in the image of God and thus worthy of acceptance. In their 1978 statement the Bishops asserted, "What individuals with disabilities need, first of all, is acceptance in this difference that can neither be denied nor overlooked. No acts of charity or justice can be of lasting value unless our actions are informed by a sincere and understanding love that penetrates the wall of strangeness and affirms the common humanity underlying all distinction. . . . Scripture teaches us that any other commandment there may be [is] all summed up in this: 'You shall love your neighbor as yourself.'(Rom. 13:9) In His wisdom, Jesus said, 'as yourself.' We must love others from the inside out, so to speak, accepting their difference from us in the same way that we accept our difference from them."[1]

An early outreach to people with disabilities, both from the Church and the State, came in the form of residential institutions for adults and children unable or unwelcome to live with their families. And while these facilities were initially developed out of concern and compassion, overcrowding, ignorance, and at times outright abuse kept many of these facilities from being truly a place to call home. When the push for deinstitutionalization happened in the late 1960s, Catholic Charities was among the first to respond. These smaller group houses, which were homes to only ten people with intellectual disabilities and their caregivers, were worlds away from the institutions in which they had previously lived. Sr. Bernadette remembers the beginning, when Catholic Charities became the third agency in New York City to receive a grant to develop group homes, and what those homes meant to people coming from large institutions: "In places like Willowbrook [a residential facility in New York State shut down after abuses and horrific living conditions were exposed], a person may be sleeping in a cot next to 99 other people. In these new homes, you have your own bedroom or shared with one other person. You eat at a table for four, instead of a hundred." And these homes not only provided humane living conditions, but a more human life. Residents left during the day for workshops or other activities, and were expected to do chores of which they were capable. "It was a real life," says Sr. Bernadette.

In addition to the physical and emotional needs of people with disabilities, the Church also recognized the need for their spiritual formation. An early pioneer in Catholic school special education was Monsignor Elmer Behrmann who founded the Department of Special Education in the Archdiocese of St. Louis in 1950. He explains, "We were pioneers in the field. In promoting the program to those in the archdiocese and beyond, we helped raise the public's awareness that children with mental disabilities had a right to a Catholic education the same as any other Catholic child." He further stated, "It's a matter of justice; it's not a matter of compassion. Justice is something you cannot deny to people."[2]

In the late 1960s and early 1970s special religious education became a formalized reality in the Catholic Church thanks to the creation of the National Apostolate for the Mentally Retarded (NAMR) and the establishment of a M.A. degree in Special Religious Education from Cardinal Stritch University in Milwaukee, WI. Graduates of this program became important ministry leaders who continue to guide this ministry today. Under the direction of Sr. Sheila Haskett and Sr. Coletta Dunn, OSF, the *Journey with Jesus* curriculum became a national teaching tool. At that time the SPRED program was created when Fr. James McCarthy and Sr. Mary Therese Harrington from the Archdiocese of Chicago began to work with parents, special educators, and catechist volunteers. SPRED continues its work in U.S. dioceses and internationally (visit *http://www.spred.org/* for more information). Many other pioneers developed curriculums in response to the concerns of parents: Sr. Helene McDonald, MHSH created lessons for sacramental preparation for the Archdiocese of Detroit; Fr. George Kuryvial, OMI developed a bible study program entitled *"Jesus Says . . ."* for the Diocese of Joliet; Sr. Marci Blum, OSF of Dubuque wrote guidelines for teaching children with learning disabilities; the Diocese of Topeka produced the REACH program; while Grace Harding of the Diocese of Pittsburgh wrote Sacramental lesson plans as well as articles for the *Catechist* magazine for several years. Many pastoral workers also developed retreat experiences, including Sr. Marge Burkle of Dubuque. All of these resources were self published and shared informally among the growing network of pastoral workers involved in this ministry, and the newly developing NAMR. In 1991, *Seasons of Grace* by Brigid O'Donnell was published by Our Sunday Visitor, and was welcomed gratefully by catechists throughout the country.

In the 1980s and 1990s, as secular educational trends moved from separate programs to "mainstreaming" and finally "inclusion," Marilyn Bishop and Patricia Carter, working from the University of Dayton became leaders in developing materials for inclusive education in Catholic schools and religious education programs. In 1996, they and the Diocese of Pittsburgh received grants from the Joseph P. Kennedy, Jr. Foundation to develop religious education curricula for students with cognitive and other disabilities. The University of Dayton's efforts produced a four-volume set for preparation for the Sacraments of Initiation focusing on individualizing lesson plans based on the various learning styles of students with disabilities. The Diocese of Pittsburgh developed the *Rose Fitzgerald Kennedy Program to Promote Catholic Education for Children and Adults with Intellectual Disabilities.* This curriculum was translated into Spanish under the guidance of Mary Brosseau of Orange County, CA. The Kennedy Foundation awarded the Diocese of Pittsburgh a grant to train catechists under the new curriculum. In all, eighty workshops were offered in dioceses and at national conferences, with over 3,000 people trained.

As demonstrated by Monsignor Behrmann, Catholic school education has also been a longtime Catholic value. The Network of Inclusive Catholic Educators, a project of the University of Dayton Institute on Pastoral Initiatives, believes in values-centered parochial school and religious education programs which acknowledge the gifts and talents of all students. Marilyn Bishop and Patricia Carter worked to create opportunities for children with disabilities to attend Catholic schools as well as religious education programs, and served as a support network and resource to individuals with disabilities and their families by providing conferences, video and print resources, consultations, workshops, and networking opportunities on the national and local level. The work continues under the leadership of Sr. Angela Ann Zukowski and Margaret Shufflebarger.

Another historic ministry was educating deaf children. As early as 1837 deaf students were being taught by religious communities. In 1853 the St. Mary's School was opened in Buffalo, and is still serving students, as are numerous other Catholic schools for the deaf throughout the United States. Among the outstanding early pioneers in deaf ministry were Mother Mary Anne Burke, CSJ, who served at St. Mary's for over sixty years; Mother Borgia Davis, CSJ, who spent her life at the St. Louis school; and Fr. Daniel Higgins, CSsR, who gave missions across North America from 1906-1959.

The first Deaf Cursillo was held in Glenview, Illinois in 1970, and has continued annually, with Cursillo number 59 held in Brooklyn, Michigan in the fall of 2005. The International Catholic Deaf Association, begun in 1949 by Deaf adults, is still going strong with sections in the United States, Canada and Venezuela. The National Catholic Office for the Deaf (NCOD) was established in 1971 during a meeting of the International Catholic Deaf Association, in recognition of the need for a national voice for the spiritual needs of Deaf Catholics and for an organization that would support pastoral workers in their services to Deaf Catholics. Its founding Executive Director, Father David Walsh, CSsR, was a fiery advocate on behalf of Catholics who were deaf or hearing impaired. Today, NCOD promotes and supports Deaf Catholic participation in the Church, and is a resource for communication, religious education, and pastoral training resources. (Visit their web site at *www.ncod.org* for a list of their resources, dates for trainings and other information.) Many deaf people are being trained for leadership roles in Ministry with the Deaf community through such programs as the Ministry Formation Program (MFP) for the Deaf in Chicago which began in 1993, and the Pastoral Ministry with the Deaf Masters Program, begun at St. Thomas University in Miami, Florida in 2001. The first three students graduated from this program in May, 2005. In addition, deaf men and women are answering the call to religious life as priests, deacons, and sisters. Fr. Thomas Coughlin, the first deaf-from-birth man to be ordained a Catholic priest in the United States is currently the director of the Dominican Missionaries for the Deaf Apostolate in the Diocese of Oakland, CA, a religious congregation of priests and brothers founded in 2004.

Along with a person's right to life and care, as well as the opportunity to grow spiritually and to use and develop one's talents, the Catholic Church clearly values community. A good example of this is seen in one early Catholic disability ministry which was, in fact, begun by and for people with disabilities. Catholics United for Spiritual Action (CUSA), a self-described apostolate of the chronically sick and disabled, was founded in 1947 by Laure Bronner, a woman who had been living in isolation for more than 45 years. CUSA is made up of small groups of people (most are Catholic, but all faiths are welcome) who encourage and support each other through letters and e-mail. Each group has an ordained priest or permanent deacon as its leader and a patron saint, motto, and spiritual orientation. They are currently planning a joint project with NCPD to reach out to veterans with disabilities returning from the wars in Iraq and Afghanistan. For further information on CUSA, visit *http:// www.cusan.org/*.

The success of CUSA underscored the idea that people with disabilities were not only to be on the *receiving* end of grace. This idea continued in the formation of the Victorious Missionaries (VM) in 1964. Victorious Missionaries' main objective was "to realize the awesome spiritual potential that people have for the Church and the World."[3] The group's founder, Fr. John Maronic asserted that "we can serve God and others in blindness, deafness, speechlessness, and even in total paralysis, provided we believe and love."[4] His Cause for Sainthood was initiated in February 2004. Chapters around the U.S. provide spiritual support to members, who participate in retreats and other activities sponsored by the national VM office headquartered at the National Shrine of Our Lady of the Snows in Belleville, IL (see *http://www. vmusa.org/*).

The late 1960s and early 1970s saw a significant growth in Catholic organizations whose sole purpose was to minister with people with disabilities, continuing the theme that people with disabilities had the right to be involved in all aspects of ministry. The National Apostolate for the Mentally Retarded (currently named the National Apostolate for Inclusion Ministry–NAfIM) was founded in 1968 by parents and pastoral workers to promote the full inclusion of persons with mental retardation in the Church community. The work of these important leaders paved the way for the *Pastoral Statement*, and the founding of NCPD. A history of this pivotal organization is detailed in the article, *The Story of the National Apostolate for Inclusion Ministry* in this volume.

The writings and insights of Jean Vanier, founder of L'Arche and Faith and Light, likewise inspired the growth of ministry with people with cognitive disabilities in the United States. Jean Vanier wrote of his experiences of bringing two young men from an institution in France to his home in Trosly. From those humble beginnings grew an international movement and network of L'Arche communities throughout the world. Preceding Vanier's work was that of Fr. Henri Bissonnier, also of France, who wrote classic books on faith formation for students with cognitive disabilities. His work was also studied by U.S. pastoral workers, and greatly influenced their ministries.

In 1975, John Keck founded a retreat program called Handicapped Encounter Christ (HEC). He recalls being invited to serve on the team for a Teens Encounter Christ (TEC) retreat. "I heard the message 'it is good to be who you are,' and immediately thought of a group of people who needed to hear this message–the children and adults with disabilities I had met as a counselor, program director, and eventually director of the Rotary Camp for Crippled Children." HEC retreats are still flourishing in numerous archdioceses and dioceses throughout the United States, including New York, Philadelphia, Boston, St. Louis, Denver, and Spokane. People with and without disabilities are enriched by this weekend retreat experience.

Catholic Charities continued its longtime work with people with blindness and visual impairments, building on the early work of the Catholic Guilds for the Blind founded in eleven dioceses between 1936 and 1957. Paul Sauerland, longtime advocate and founding NCPD board member, remembers the early days of the Catholic Guilds in Brooklyn. "We would arrange to hold our meetings right after the secular American Association of Workers for the Blind meetings," he laughs. "We'd try to grab up members that way." The Guild's main emphasis then was "to promote the spiritual, mental, moral and physical welfare of blind or partially blind persons by sponsoring and conducting religious, recreational, welfare and social rehabilitation, and guidance programs for said blind persons."[5] In 1984 a national organization, the Catholic Association of Persons with Visual Impairment (CAPVI) was founded under the leadership of Monsignor Paul Lackner, to promote the delivery of services to Catholics who are blind or visually impaired. Among their achievements was production of a video entitled *Late Afternoon Workers*. In 2002, CAPVI merged with NCPD in order to more effectively advance their goals. The Monsignor Paul Lackner Fund was established to support access initiatives for Catholics with visual impairments. A current NCPD project utilizing this Fund is the production of the Catholic Lectionary and Sacramentary in three sizes of large print for distribution to priests and lay Catholics.

CONNECTING NATIONALLY
WITH THE U.S. CATHOLIC BISHOPS

In 1973, NCOD made a request to become a formal part of the United States Catholic Conference (USCC). This request was denied, as the bishops felt it a mistake to single out one group of people with a disability for a national office. However, in 1975, the USCC invited leaders in disability ministry to serve on a National Advisory Committee on Ministry with Handicapped Persons. From this Committee came the drafting of the 1978 *Pastoral Statement of U.S. Catholic Bishops on People with Disabilities.* This document would prove groundbreaking. The Bishops made a provocative and compelling case for the move from charitable works for Catholics with disabilities to their full inclusion in all aspects of both Church and national life. They wrote: "It is not enough merely to affirm the rights of people with disabilities. We must actively work to make them real in the fabric of modern society . . . [the Church] must work to increase the public's sensitivity toward the needs of people with disabilities and support their rightful demand for justice."[6] The *Pastoral Statement* made it clear that people with disabilities had not only rights within the Church, the right to religious education, the sacraments, access to church buildings and programs, but the right to a welcoming attitude from their fellow Christians: "If people with disabilities are to become equal partners in the Christian community, injustices must be eliminated and ignorance and apathy replaced by increased sensitivity and warm acceptance."[7] The Bishops made clear that the inclusion of people with disabilities was to be *full* participation: " . . . they have the same duty as all members of the community to do the Lord's work in the world, according to their God-given talents and capacity. Because individuals may not be fully aware of the contribution they can make, Church leaders should consult with them, offering suggestions on practical ways of serving."[8]

The call was made. The practical implications of this call, however, were long-reaching and needed concrete implementation. The same Advisory Committee which had been influential in the drafting of the 1978 *Pastoral Statement* secured funds from the American Board of Catholic Missions (ABCM) to open the National Catholic Office for Persons with Disabilities (now the National Catholic Partnership on Disability–NCPD). The office opened in 1982 and had as its mission the further implementation of the directives of the *Pastoral Statement*, which insists that disabled Catholics must be able to participate in the celebrations and obligations of their faith. The office would support diocesan directors in their efforts to create access, providing training, creating resources, and holding workshops and conferences.

NCPD's first board of directors was composed of the Executive Committee of that initial Advisory Committee and was headed by Monsignor Thomas Cribbin of Brooklyn Catholic Charities. Founding members included representatives from NAfIM (Br. Joseph Moloney, OSF), NCOD (Rev. David Walsh), SPRED (Sr. Mary Therese Harrington), Paul Sauerland, representing the concerns of Catholics with visual impairments, and nearly a dozen other pastoral workers and Catholics with disabilities. Dr. David Byers served the board as the liaison to the U.S. Catholic bishops' conference. He had been instrumental in securing the funds from the ABCM. An early action of NCPD's board was to hire Sister Rita Baum, SSJ as the organization's first executive director. Sr. Rita had been the director of the program for the deaf in the Diocese of St. Augustine and more recently the director of the Diocesan Office for the Handicapped. The NCPD office officially opened on August 15, 1982, in Washington, D.C., with a staff of two: Sr. Rita and her associate, Janice Benton, who had served two years on the Advisory Committee.

The early years at NCPD found Sr. Rita on the road much of the time, traveling to meet with bishops and offering training and support to diocesan and parish personnel, many of whom had been laboring in their dioceses for years. Where there were diocesan ministries, it was found that they were situated in a wide range of offices including education, religious education, Catholic Charities, and Family Life. This differentiation of placement of diocesan disability ministry continues to this day. NCPD also hosted national conferences, including a retreat in Jacksonville, FL as well as a series of regional meetings. Groundwork was laid for what would become the *Guidelines for the Celebration of the Sacraments for Persons with Disabilities* approved by the bishops in 1995. NCPD published the first edition of the groundbreaking *Opening Doors to Persons with Disabilities*, Volumes I and II in 1985, and updated and revised it a decade later. This resource serves as a guidebook for developing ministry programs, and provides ministry models, bishops' documents, essays, access surveys, and fact sheets. Topics covered include universal design, education, ethics, and family support.

The work of NCPD, while clearly focused on change within the Church, also had impact on the national scene. During NCPD's Tenth Anniversary Report to the U.S. Catholic Bishops in 1992, NCPD Board member Most Reverend Francis E. George, then Bishop of Yakima, highlighted the civil impact of the religious office: "NCPD has also used the 1978 *Pastoral Statement* as a foundation from which to press for civil legislation which opens previously closed doors in the general society, thereby fostering greater participation in public life on the part of citizens with disabilities. The greatest success in this venture has been the 1990 landmark Americans With Disabilities Act . . . this law sets out patterns and means for helping people with disabilities become functional in situations which previously handicapped them."[9] Indeed a quotation from the *Pastoral Statement* included in a letter of support for the bill from the USCC was read on the floor of Congress by Senator Tom Harkin as he introduced the Americans with Disabilities Act with these words: "Defense of the right to life implies the defense of other rights which enable the individual with a disability to achieve the fullest measure of personal development. . . . These include the right to equal opportunity in education, in employment, in housing, as well as the right to free access to public accommodations, facilities and services. Passage of this bill will mean discrimination solely on the basis of handicaps will be not only immoral but illegal." NCPD worked with an interfaith committee called together by the National Organization on Disability (NOD) to publish a guide on the moral and legal responsibility of faith communities under the ADA. The Catholic version of the guide is available through NCPD under the title of *A Loving Justice.*

In May of 1991, Mary Jane Owen assumed the position of NCPD's executive director. Herself a woman with multiple disabilities, she brought a different perspective and new insight to leadership at NCPD. She spoke from a powerful place about the reality of disability, saying that "disabilities are the normal expected and anticipated outcome of the risks, stresses and strains of the living process itself. Disability is not something that happens only to the unlucky few but is an event that can be anticipated by us all." With those simple sentences, Owen broke down the walls between "us and them," between those who currently live with disabilities and those who do not. She awakened in the people who read her words and heard her speak a consciousness of the fact that, indeed, we all are dependant upon one another, in ways we might not have thought about previously. And that dependency, in a culture that worships the rugged individual, is in fact something to be celebrated. In her article, "The Rich Tapestry of Life and Disability,"[10] Owen quotes Pope John Paul II to underscore this point: "We, the disabled people of the world, must illustrate and teach the people of Christ's Church the power of the powerless, the strength of our shared vulnerability, the wisdom of the concrete-minded, the beauty to be glimpsed beyond sight, the healing words not spoken aloud." And in her own words: "Our vulnerability, which has been encoded into our gene pool, is the catalyst which brings us into community and the Church with renewed recognition that we need each other and Our Lord."

At an international conference on disability hosted by the Vatican in November 1992, Owen made the point again and again that a culture of radical individualism is not only dangerous to our physical lives, but to our spiritual lives as well: "Without awareness of our mutual interdependence, we may mistake our temporary personal independence as the source of our power."[11]

Along with the important insight that there is great wisdom in vulnerability, Owen also provided a much-needed intellectual and spiritual link between the disability rights movement and the work of the pro-life community. Discussing the phrase, "I'd rather be dead than disabled," Owen writes: "Whether a given eugenics campaign endorses euthanasia, infanticide, or abortion, those less devoted to our belief in the sanctity of life are easy prey to each retelling of those ancient and no longer appropriate terrors of dependency which stalked the nightmares of our ancestors. The assaults upon life move forward because so few of us are knowledgeable or comfortable enough to speak out positively about the power of the powerless and the potential of those who are disabled."[12]

Throughout the Millennium Year, Catholics throughout the world celebrated Vatican-proclaimed Jubilee Days. December 3, 2000 was declared the Jubilee Day for People with Disabilities. In recognition of this day, the Vatican issued a series of important statements relating to people with disabilities. Pope John Paul II's address on that day opened with the following challenge: "This afternoon's celebration shows that the integration of disabled persons has made progress, even though there is still a long way to go; indeed, there are some important and urgent needs on which it would be good to pause and reflect. First of all, the right that every disabled man and woman has in any country of the world to a dignified life. It is not only a question of satisfying their specific needs, but even more of seeing their own desire for acceptance and autonomy recognized. Integration must become an attitude and a culture; at the same time, lawmakers and government leaders must give their consistent support to this cause."[13] Excerpts from this and other statements surrounding this Jubilee Day can be found at the following link to NCPD's web site: *http://www.ncpd.org/vatican_statements.htm*

In May of 2004, Janice Benton, who had helped to build the office, working on staff since its opening in 1982, assumed the title of Executive Director of NCPD. Her 25 years of experience in disability advocacy, strong focus, and longtime passion for this ministry brought yet another valuable perspective to the leadership of the office. She notes that the real strength of NCPD is its national network of diocesan directors of disability ministry, and its ability to reach out to partners, both raising awareness and then providing the resources and training to support the work necessary to further implement the 1978 *Pastoral Statement*. A further strength is its ability to be flexible and see things from different perspectives while still keeping its eye on the ultimate goal of the spiritual nurture of Catholics with disabilities by advancing their inclusion in Church and society. An early mission of NCPD was to establish a separate office of disability ministry in each diocese. Years later, while revising the resource *Opening Doors*, she and the writing committee saw that other models could work. They advised that it's possible to have a diocesan consultant whose job it is to work with all of the other diocesan offices on disability issues because all aspects of diocesan life, regardless of the office, have areas in which disability awareness is crucial.

Ms. Benton sees as very important her role as support person for diocesan directors of disability offices because it is the diocesan directors and advocates in parishes, working *with* Catholics with disabilities and family members who can create the access and inclusion needed in each parish. Since a diocesan director's job is so daunting, she encourages them to delegate responsibilities and to network with their colleagues in other diocesan offices.

In addition to its mission being grounded in the implementation of the 1978 *Pastoral Statement*, NCPD promotes the *Guidelines for the Celebration of the Sacraments with Persons with Disabilities*, approved by the U.S. bishops in June 1995. These guidelines provide pastoral guidance on sacramental access for people with disabilities. In 2003 the office partnered with the Publications Office of the USCCB to release a parish resource guide for the inclusion of persons with disabilities in various aspects of parish life, *Opening Doors of Welcome and Justice to Parishioners with Disabilities*, which is available at their website (*www.usccb.org*). NCPD advocates on legislative issues which impact the lives of people with disabilities, including education, health care, life issues, social security reform, and transportation. Each year NCPD cosponsors with the USCCB Office of Social Development and World Peace, and a number of other national organizations, the national conference of Catholic social justice directors from dioceses throughout the U.S., infusing a disability perspective into the issues addressed at the gathering.

COLLABORATIVE EFFORTS

Over the years, NCPD has engaged in a number of collaborative ventures with ministry partners, including the publication of *A Loving Justice* and co-sponsorship of the annual social justice gathering described above. Each year, in conjunction with the Community Partnership Program of the National Organization on Disability they sponsor an Opening Doors Award contest, providing $1,000 to the winning diocesan or parish programs.

In 1991, NCPD co-sponsored a national gathering at the Catholic University of America in Washington, DC with NAfIM, which brought together Catholics with disabilities, family members, NAfIM members, diocesan directors, and other pastoral workers to network, share resources, and learn from experts in the field. Additional collaborative efforts include serving on the boards of interfaith ministries such as Pathways to Promise (an outreach ministry to people with mental illness) and the Committee on Disabilities of the National Council of Churches.

NEW REALITIES

Much has changed in society and in the Church since the first Catholic residential schools were opened for students who were deaf, blind, or cognitively disabled. The advent of federal and state laws protecting the rights of people with disabilities to education, employment, housing, and public accommodations has heightened expectations for access and inclusion in faith communities. No longer are people content to be occasional participants in parish life, or the recipients of a well-meaning but misguided ministry "to" them. The emphasis now is on inclusion, leadership, and self-direction. As evidenced by the Catholic Deaf community and many diocesan directors of disability ministry, more and more people with disabling conditions are taking leadership roles in creating and promoting accessible communities of faith.

Another reality within the Catholic Church is the closing or consolidation of ministry offices. Securing sufficient funding is an ongoing challenge calling for creativity and collaboration.

FUTURE DIRECTIONS AND INITIATIVES

As NCPD approaches its 25th anniversary in light of these new realities, it moves forward on a number of projects, and anticipates new directions. NCPD will continue its outreach to diocesan and parish disability directors, and partner organizations, and will utilize technology to increase and facilitate communication through web forums and conferencing. It will continue to work collaboratively with its many ministry partners, including NAfIM, NCOD, CUSA, HEC, and the Victorious Missionaries to further their mutual ministry goals. It will also continue to co-sponsor conferences with national partners, and will consider new ways of sharing resources. It will focus new attention on the needs of people with brain injury and multiple chemical sensitivities.

NCPD is working on an *Access Manual for Catholic Facilities*, which will provide specific access guidelines and architectural drawings, as well as a photo sampling of "Access Dos and Don'ts." It is also in the process of expanding its web site (*www.ncpd.org*) to provide updated resources and links to partners and other relevant organizations. In response to concerns voiced by people with disabilities and family members, NCPD will establish National Catholic Task Forces on several issues, including mental illness and inclusive Catholic education.

CONCLUSION

The journey is far from over. For all of those people who live safely in smaller group homes, there are many more that left institutions with nowhere to go. Some diocesan or parish leaders still have little awareness of the very real needs of people with disabilities in their parishes and communities. Financial support of disability ministries is an ongoing concern. But the call put out in 1978 is still strong. In a follow-up to the Pastoral Statement, the U.S. Bishops in 1998 issued a Statement entitled *Welcome and Justice for Persons with Disabilities: A Framework of Access and Inclusion*. In this Statement, the Bishops remind us of the principles of justice and inclusion that were the framework for their initial letter. Along with the rights of people with disabilities to life and equal opportunity, "we must recognize and appreciate the contribution persons with disabilities can make to the Church's spiritual life, and encourage them to do the Lord's work in the world according to their God-given talents and capacity."[14]

Because, in truth, "We are a single flock under the care of a single shepherd. There can be no separate Church for people with disabilities."[15]

NOTES

1. National Conference of Catholic Bishops. *Pastoral Statement of U.S. Catholic Bishops on People with Disabilities*, rev. ed. Washington, DC: United States Catholic Conference, 1989, par. 3. The original version of this *Pastoral Statement*, published November 16, 1978, was revised in 1989 to update language used in referring to people with disabilities.

2. Schildz, Jean M. "Special education department celebrates 50 years." St. Louis, MO: St. Louis Review Online, October 20, 2000. *http://www.stlouisreview.com/archive/archive.php?page=001020_03.shtml*

3. Who Are the VMs? *http://www.vmusa.org/who.htm*

4. Reck, Carleen. *Able to Uplift*. Belleville, IL: Missionary Oblates of Mary Immaculate Publishing, page 9.

5. Sauerland, Paul Joseph. *Catholic Guilds for the Blind in the United States: A Survey of Eleven Diocesan Agencies for the Blind, 1936-1959*. Master's Dissertation, Fordham University School of Social Services, New York, 1959.

6. National Conference of Catholic Bishops. *Pastoral Statement of U.S. Catholic Bishops on People with Disabilities*, rev. ed. Washington, DC: United States Catholic Conference, 1989, par. 11.

7. Ibid, par. 13.

8. Ibid, par. 17.

9. George, Most Rev. Francis. "NCPD's Tenth Anniversary Report to U.S. Catholic Bishops" in *Opening Doors to People with Disabilities, Volume I: Pastoral Manual*. Washington, DC: National Catholic Office for Persons with Disabilities, 1995, page 162.

10. Owen, Mary Jane. "The Rich Tapestry of Life and Disability" in *The Priest*. Huntington, IN: Our Sunday Visitor, Vol. 59, No. 7, July 2003, page 10.

11. Owen, Mary Jane. "The Wisdom of Human Vulnerability, Disability: A Tie Which Binds" presented at the Seventh International Conference, *Your Members Are the Body of Christ, Persons with Disabilities in Society*, Vatican City, November 19-2,1992.

12. Owen, Mary Jane. "Frayed At the Edges: The Intertwined Threads of Life and Disability," in Respect Life Program Packet, NCCB Secretariat for Pro-Life Activities. Washington, DC: United States Catholic Conference, 1993.

13. Pope John Paul II. *Jubilee of the Disabled, Address of John Paul II*, Vatican City, December 3, 2000. *http://www.vatican.va/holy_father/john_paul_ii/speeches/documents/hf_jp-ii_spe_20001203_jubildisabled_en.html*

14. United States Catholic Conference. "Welcome and Justice for Persons with Disabilities: A Framework of Access and Inclusion." Washington, DC: United States Catholic Conference, 1998, par. 7.

15. United States Catholic Conference. "Welcome and Justice for Persons with Disabilities: A Framework of Access and Inclusion" Washington, DC: United States Catholic Conference, 1998, par 1.

The Story of the National Apostolate for Inclusion Ministry

Barbara J. Lampe, JD

SUMMARY. The work of the National Apostolate for Inclusion Ministry is reflected in its Mission Statement–Called together by our baptism as persons with and without Mental Retardation and proclaiming and witnessing to the Good News that all persons are created in God's image and likeness as proclaimed by the teachings of the Catholic Church, we the members of the National Apostolate for Inclusion Ministry promote the full inclusion of persons with Mental Retardation and welcome their gifts into the Body of Christ. *[Article copies available for a fee from The Haworth Document Delivery Service: 1-800-HAWORTH. E-mail address: <docdelivery@haworthpress.com> Website: <http://www.HaworthPress.com> © 2006 by The Haworth Press, Inc. All rights reserved.]*

KEYWORDS. Disability, mental retardation, Catholic Church, inclusion, apostolate

---

Barbara J. Lampe is a mother, attorney, disability activist, writer and Executive Director of the National Apostolate for Inclusion Ministry.

[Haworth co-indexing entry note]: "The Story of the National Apostolate for Inclusion Ministry." Lampe, Barbara J. Co-published simultaneously in *Journal of Religion, Disability & Health* (The Haworth Pastoral Press, an imprint of The Haworth Press, Inc.) Vol. 10, No. 1/2, 2006, pp. 55-74; and: *Disability Advocacy Among Religious Organizations: Histories and Reflections* (ed: Albert A. Herzog, Jr.) The Haworth Pastoral Press, an imprint of The Haworth Press, Inc., 2006, pp. 55-74. Single or multiple copies of this article are available for a fee from The Haworth Document Delivery Service [1-800-HAWORTH, 9:00 a.m. - 5:00 p.m. (EST). E-mail address: docdelivery@haworthpress.com].

Available online at http://www.haworthpress.com/web/JRDH
© 2006 by The Haworth Press, Inc. All rights reserved.
doi:10.1300/J095v10n01_05

INTRODUCTION

The story of the National Apostolate for Inclusion Ministry describes some of the struggle for the just valuation of people with an intelligence quotient of less than 70 in the Catholic Church in the United States.

Things have turned 180° in the minds of some Catholics. This became clear to me not too long ago as I was teaching a seventh grade religious education class on Jesus the Way. Since I accepted all persons with disabilities into my class, Julita (not her real name), a young teenage girl with severe cognitive disabilities, was brought to my class midway in February. She was quiet and charming. I usually had some activity or picture pages for her to illustrate what the rest of the class was doing. When I asked a question, she would often raise her hand, and I would call on her even though she did not speak.

Shortly thereafter, her mother told me that her daughter would be receiving the Sacrament of Confirmation in May. I was stunned. It is the practice in our diocese for persons to receive this Sacrament in the eighth grade after two years of preparation. She had been placed in the seventh grade where no final preparation for Confirmation was taking place. When I spoke to the director of religious education (DRE) about this, I was told that because of her mental condition, there was no need to provide formation for the Sacrament, since she would not be tested on prayers, the commandments, gifts of the Holy Spirit, the corporal and spiritual works of mercy, etc. Thus, it did not matter that she was being rushed to Confirmation. She had been placed in my class because the eighth grade teacher could not deal with her.

My concerns about treating her differently, placing her cold into a group of teens that she did not know, for a ceremony that would surely be a mystery to her fell on deaf ears. The DRE had already promised her mother that she would receive the Sacrament in a few months. I jeopardized my good relationship with the DRE by bringing the matter to the pastor, insisting that my student needed to receive Confirmation with the new seventh grade community in which she had established herself, and that she needed time to develop her own spiritual responses on her way to fuller Church membership. The pastor must have agreed with me, because she received the Sacrament of Confirmation a year later.

Forty years ago, Julita would not have made it into my classroom, much less to the chair of the Bishop confirming a group of young people with the oil of Confirmation. Her parents would have been ashamed to bring her to Mass, but if she did attend the Sacred Liturgy, she would not have been allowed to join her fellow parishioners at the Eucharistic

Table. Now, apparently, some Catholic religious educators have come
to think that persons who are mentally retarded, with intellectual or cognitive disabilities (or whatever term now serves as less offensive), do
not need any spiritual nourishing or community awareness at all for the
reception of the Sacraments.

Today, Julita, may receive religious formation either by being included in a religious education class or by attending a special religious
education class, may be individually prepared to receive the Sacraments
of Initiation and may be involved in a parish ministry such as handing
out bulletins, but she would not be accepted in a Catholic school or on a
parish, archdiocesan or bishops' conference committee. If she is in a
parish with a SPRED program or a Faith and Light group she may have
some opportunity to celebrate faith based activities with peers with and
without disabilities.

VATICAN II

Revolutionary changes in how the Catholic Church perceives the liturgy, the laity and the world in which it dwells flow from the council of
Catholic bishops known as Vatican II (1962-1965). For our purposes
here, the post-conciliar understanding of the individual and his or her
place in the liturgy will be addressed briefly.

The Constitution on the Sacred Liturgy, *Sacrosanctum Consilium*,
was issued December 4, 1963. This was the very first document issued
by the Council. The Council fathers rejected the passivity in the pews
that had characterized the Latin Mass and set out, in numerous para-
graphs, a reconstituted liturgy in which all the faithful take part "fully
aware of what they are doing, actively engaged in the rite and enriched
by it" (Vatican II, *Sacrosantum Concillium*, paragraph 11). The document on the Eucharist (S.C.R., *Eucharisticum Mysterium*, 25 May,
1967) instructs that the Lord is present to His Church in liturgical celebrations in the body of the faithful gathered in His name, in His Word
(Holy Scripture), the ministry of the priest, and His presence under the
species of bread and wine (Paragraph 9). In The Dogmatic Constitution
on the Church (Vatican II, *Lumen Gentium*, 21 November, 1964), another very early document of the council, Chapter IV on the Laity perti-
nently states in paragraph 32, "In the Church not everyone marches
along the same path, yet all are called to sanctity and have obtained an
equal privilege of faith through the justice of God (cf. 2 Pet.1: 1)."

THE BEGINNING OF AN APOSTOLATE

There was something in the air, but the effects had not yet been felt. So, it was probably not coincidental that in 1961, Catholic teachers of religion in the United States, at that time mostly priests and members of religious orders, spoke publicly for the first time about their feelings of inadequacy and isolation in their diocesan programs or private apostolates for persons with mental retardation. They were outraged that children and adults were excluded from full participation at Eucharist and other sacraments because of their cognitive and intellectual abilities. Their voices rose at the Inter-American Confraternity of Christian Doctrine (CCD or currently termed religious education) Congress held in Dallas, Texas in December 1961.[1]

Within the then National Conference of Diocesan Directors (NCDD) there was formed the National CCD Apostolate for the Mentally Retarded to promote religious instruction for mentally retarded persons. A follow-up to the Dallas meeting was scheduled for January 15-16, 1962. Here aims and purposes, ideas about teacher training, parish centers and institutions were discussed.[2] However, the broader concern for parish inclusion and hospitality made it clear that the NCDD structure was not appropriate.[3]

Again at the CCD Congress in Pittsburgh in September 1966, the 500 delegates attending special sessions on religious education for persons with mental retardation enthusiastically affirmed the idea for a national apostolate to honor their rights as people of God. A committee formed to continue the work, conducted a survey among diocesan directors of religious education in the spring of 1967 inquiring among other things whether religious education programs existed in their diocese, whether they were interested in forming such programs and whether they would cooperate in a National Apostolate for this purpose. When 97 of 150 responded in the affirmative, a business meeting and conference was held August 25-28 in West Hartford, Connecticut, establishing National Apostolate with Mental Retardation (NAMR).

This august body of founders included Rev. Matt Pesaniello, president, of Newark, Rev. Joseph A. Goebel, vice-president, of Cleveland, Sr. Mary John Minetta SHF (author of the first catechetical text for the reception of First Holy Communion for children with mental retardation), Secretary, of Los Angeles, Mrs. Marvin Crull, Treasurer, of Pittsburgh, Rev. Cal Gengras of Connecticut, Rev. Gerard Sabourin of Rhode Island, Rev. Bob Wagner of Massachusetts, Sr. Mary Therese Harrington (one of the founders of the SPRED program in Chicago), Sr.

Sheila Haskett, OSF (St. Coletta School, Jefferson, Wisconsin), Sr. Dolores Wilson, SND de N (Lt. Joseph P. Kennedy Institute, Washington, DC), Sr. Maxine Kraemer, RSCJ (St. Madeleine Sophie's Training Center, El Cajon, California), Rev. Ron Gilmore and Sr. Veronice Born, CSJ, both of Wichita, Mrs. Robert McClinton of Colorado Springs, and Marie Stengel of Buffalo.[4]

CHANGES IN NAME

The National Apostolate has changed its name three times in its nearly forty-year history. In the beginning, the name was National Apostolate for the Mentally Retarded (NAMR). In the mid-seventies, there arose a movement to change the name. There was a feeling that the existing name did not give proper dignity to the people with whom the Apostolate's members were sharing their lives. In 1978, Sr. Sheila Haskett, OSF, became president at the meeting where the name was changed to National Apostolate with Mentally Retarded Persons (NAMRP). She said, "Our special people seem so gifted in their ability to make other people feel that they are worthwhile and important. They uplift and build with their simple affection and expressions of caring and esteem. I have long studied this beautiful gift, prayed to acquire it and tried to emulate it. But it is a steep road to climb."[5]

On August 4, 1992 at the Denver meeting, the membership again voted to change the name of the organization, this time to National Apostolate with People with Mental Retardation (NAPMR). Then Board President, Jill Johnson, explained the meaning of the changes. The word *people* is placed before *mental retardation* because the focus of NAPMR is on the people, not on their disability. The word *people* seemed to invoke more importance than the word *persons*. The term *apostolate* was retained because it suggested affinity with Jesus and his apostles. The term *with* remained because the Apostolate is not a ministry for people but has mutuality, that is we minister to each other.[6]

The last name change to National Apostolate for Inclusion Ministry was adopted by the membership through ballot and phone poll in the summer of 1997. "The new name reflects that we are an Apostolate, that is, a lay ministry which supports the work of our Church. Our ministry is to include all people in the Catholic Church. Specifically, we share the journey of persons with mental retardation in the life of our Catholic Church."[7]

Most recently, at its 2005 Summer Board Meeting in Mobile, the board of directors amended its tag line from "Supporting the Inclusion of Persons with Mental Retardation in the Catholic Church" to "Promoting the Full Participation of Persons with Intellectual Disabilities in the Life of the Catholic Church."

HAPPENING IN THE SIXTIES

The didactic method of Catholic religious education in the United States would take a momentous turn after the publication of *Modern Catechetics–Message and Method in Religious Formation* (McMillan, 1962) edited by Catholic University professor and priest, Rev. Gerard S. Sloyan. The story of God, Jesus, breaking into history should be told in parts and completely "in such a way that it opens up to the student the possibility of response in terms of decision, commitment, and faith."[8] In time the acronym CCD would be replaced with the terms religious education, catechist (the teacher who hands on the tradition) and catechesis (sharing the teaching of Christ).

Other major events having an impact on the emergence of the Apostolate were: (1) the National Catholic Education Association (NCEA) began publishing a directory of special facilities and programs for handicapped children and adults; (2) the convening of a blue ribbon panel by President John F. Kennedy in 1961, which by presidential order in 1966 by President Lyndon B. Johnson became the President's Committee on Mental Retardation; and (3) September 30, 1968, when the US Congress passed PL 90-538, Handicapped Children's Early Education Assistance Act authorizing grants for programs in preschool and early education programs for handicapped children.

EARLY DAYS OF THE APOSTOLATE

The new Apostolate hit the ground running far ahead of the rush to come. The first quarterly was published in September 1968; the first newsletter "Newslites" edited by Father Bob Wagner came out in March 1972. Joyful that they at last had a community, the members grew by leaps and bounds.

The Quarterly, first edited by Father Matt Pesaniello was full of articles of success stories, outlines for success, diocesan programs, homilies, resources, and reflections, often presented at NAMR conferences, by such icons as Père Henri Bissonier, Stanley Hauerwas, Sr. Mary Theodore Hegeman, OSF, Robert Perske, Jean Vanier, and Wolf Wolfensberger, writings by cardinals, archbishops, bishops, priests, religious, parents, educators, and academicians too numerous to name but each worthy contributors to the movement in their own right. Although the bishops of the United States had not spoken formally on disability, there were dioceses such the Archdiocese of Atlanta that developed a comprehensive statement on Catholics with mental retardation.[9]

HAPPENING IN THE SEVENTIES

The Vatican issued the *General Directory on Catechesis* in 1971. Subsequently, the National Conference of Catholic Bishops issued a number of important documents relating to Christian education. The first document was *To Teach as Jesus Did: A Pastoral Message on Catholic Education*, NCCB, November 1972. In this document the bishops described three interlocking dimensions of message, fellowship and service. The next was *Sharing the Light of Faith: National Catechetical Directory for Catholics of the United States*, NCCB, 1979.

On December 7, 1976, the US Bishops created an Advisory Committee on Ministry to the Handicapped. In 1979, as a bow to NAMRP's name change, the committee was renamed Advisory Committee on Ministry with Handicapped Persons.

The hopes of NAMR and NAMRP for their Church to address issues important to all persons with disabilities came to fruition when the US bishops issued *Pastoral Statement of U.S. Bishops on Handicapped People* on November 16, 1978.

Geraldo Rivera received national attention for his 1972 news stories on the abuse of mentally retarded patients at Staten Island's Willowbrook State School for WABC in New York. The incident provoked a renewed emphasis on closing large institutions.

In 1975, the US Congress passed Public Law 94-142, Education for All Handicapped Children Act. Funds were provided to all jurisdictions that assured a free and appropriate public education (FAPE) in the least restrictive environment (LRE).

EARLY YEARS OF THE APOSTOLATE

The Apostolate held its first annual conference in West Hartford in August 1970 with the theme "The Spiritual Equality of All God's Children." From then on, the Quarterly publication tended to reflect conference themes as well as concerns with special religious education.[10] Rev. Edmund S. Borycz served as editor from 1974 to 1980.

Trinity College provided space for the first national office. Rev. Bob Malloy, OFM Cap as the first executive director in 1973 took responsibility for issuing the newsletter monthly beginning in 1974 and facilitated the incorporation of NAMR as a nonprofit organization.[11] Beginning in 1974, board officers changed each year. Brother Joe Moloney of Brooklyn followed him in office as executive director in 1977, and subsequently moved the office to Brooklyn.

While the Apostolate was not an official agency of the US Bishops Conference, nevertheless, there was much interaction with their offices. Apostolate members were on the Bishops' Advisory Committee. The Apostolate submitted thirteen items for inclusion in the national catechetical directory, *Sharing the Light of Faith*.[12] The following members were on the committee that drafted the Bishops' pastoral letter on the handicapped: Father Thomas Cribbin (Chair), Father John Aurelio, Mrs. Fran Campbell, Father Bob Malloy, and Sr. Mary Therese Harrington.

As early as 1975, NAMR members called for the establishment of a national catholic office to serve all persons with disabilities. In 1977, a resolution was passed at the conference in San Diego that each diocese or archdiocese in the United States equip at least one parish in each deanery with architectural modifications to serve persons with physical disabilities and that each parish begin to remove all barriers that hinder persons with disabilities from full participation in parish life.[13] Perhaps most importantly, the membership passed a resolution in 1979 recommending that NAMRP provide national leadership to work toward obtaining an "approval for handicapped persons, regardless of the severity of their disabilities, to celebrate the Sacraments of Christian Initiation as full participating members of God's Church."[14] (In the Catholic Church, Sacraments of Initiation are Baptism, Confirmation and Eucharist.)

During this time, NAMR/NAMRP began to be recognized as a force for the promotion of the dignity and rights of persons with mental retardation. Numerous invitations came to the members of the organization from both Catholic and secular venues. For example, in 1979, executive director, Br. Joe Moloney reported attending the following meetings: Advisory Committee on Ministry with Handicapped Persons, NCEA Convention and executive committee meeting, AAMD Meeting, Open Doors Conference and speaking at the Catholic Hospital Convention. There was official national involvement in preparing for the International Year of Disabled Persons announced in 1979 for 1981.

Virginia Kreyer of the National Council of Churches of Christ invited Br. Joe Moloney, a Franciscan in Brooklyn, to the Committee on Disabilities because the Apostolate was doing "neat things." The committee had also reached out to a number of groups that were not members, including the Missouri Synod (Lutheran).[15]

The Apostolate newsletters reflected commentary on the Bishop's Pastoral Statement. There was some concern that the statement was not strong enough in its language rejecting programs that isolate persons with certain disabilities. Moreover, the statement could be construed as ambiguous on the issue of including persons with disabilities in the sacred liturgy, in the Sacraments of Eucharist, Confirmation, Penance, Matrimony, or Holy Orders.

The theme of the 1979 conference was "Parish Awareness–Reaching Out–Receiving," reflecting a growing frustration with the lack of hospitality for people with mental retardation at the parish level. At this conference, a parish awareness program was distributed. "Special to God, Special to Us" was a filmstrip accompanied by a script; over 400 sets were sold in six months. It also was the beginning of a number of subsequent annual conferences by the Apostolate where the organization attempted to realize the intent of the Bishops' Pastoral Statement.

Volume 17 of the 1979 Edition of the New Catholic Encyclopedia included the article "National Apostolate for the Mentally Retarded (NAMR)" written by Brother Joseph Moloney.

HAPPENING IN THE EIGHTIES

The declaration of the United Nations establishing an International Year of Disabled Persons in 1981 brought about great public awareness of barriers facing all persons with disabilities. The United States government created a committee to address the issues of the International Year of the Disabled Person with sixteen cabinet level representatives and nine government agency representatives. Sr. Suzanne SND de N, executive director, NCEA Department of Special Education was an official "partner." The National Organization on Disability (NOD), a private, nonprofit organization was established to succeed the US Council for the International Year of Disabled Persons through the Decade of Disabled Persons (1983-1992).

The United States Postal Service issued a ten-cent stamp commemorating mental retardation. In 1987, the American Association on Mental Deficiency (AAMD) changed its name to American Association on Mental Retardation.

The Vatican issued *Document of the Holy See for the International Year of Disabled Persons: To All Who Work for the Disabled*, March 4, 1981. The document stated, "(S)haring by the disabled in the life of society must be inspired by the principles of integration, normalization and personalization" (Paragraph 4). The document also stated, "(T)he disabled person must be urged not to be content with being only the subject of rights, accustomed to receiving care and solidarity from others, with a merely passive attitude. He is not only a receiver; he must be helped to be a giver to the full extent of his capabilities. An important and decisive moment in his formation will be reached when he becomes aware of his dignity and worth and recognizes that something is expected from him, and that he, too, can and should contribute to the progress and well-being of his family and community. The idea that he has of himself should, of course, be realistic, but also positive, allowing him to see himself as a person capable of responsibility, able to exercise his own will and to collaborate with others" (Paragraph 12).

The Holy Father Pope John Paul II celebrated the feast of Corpus Christi (The Feast of the Body and Blood of Christ) in 1981 with and for the handicapped people in Rome, thus creating a model still followed by some of his fellow bishops. About this time, the National Conference of Catholic Charities adopted a policy statement on persons with handicapping conditions or disabilities. The USCC Advisory Committee on Ministry with Handicapped People sponsored a meeting for those named as diocesan disability ministry coordinators. The Rev. Harold Wilke gave the opening address.

The early dream of the Apostolate, articulated as early as 1976, for a national Catholic office concerned with persons with all disabilities was realized in 1982, when the U.S. Bishops created the National Catholic Office with Persons with Disabilities.

The Code of Canon Law was revised in 1983. There was some feeling among disability advocates that there was discrimination against disabled persons.

MIDDLE YEARS OF THE APOSTOLATE

Br. Joe Moloney was allowed by his religious order to serve as executive director for nine years. During his tenure, the membership (the Apostolate is a membership organization) grew to over 1,000 members across the United States. A number of members developed useful materials, such as the resource booklet developed by Sr. Bernadette Webber (Diocese of St. Cloud), a two-year project. Sr. Gabrielle Kowalski OFS (Professor, Cardinal Stritch College) became editor of the newsletter and she continued the publishing of information from sacred and secular sources as well as instituting opinion articles and a greater number of letters to the editor. In addition several helpful brochures were published.

In 1980, Br. Joe appeared on television with Sr. Bernadette Downs, NAMRP president. He reported with some astonishment that he was presented the key to the City of Green Bay shortly after the annual meeting at which the Apostolate had become a partner in the IYDP (International Year of the Disabled Persons).[16]

In 1981, gifted author and educator, Sr. Sheila Haskett OSF, became the editor of the NAMRP Quarterly Publication. Sr. Coletta Dunn OSF assisted her. The Quarterlies during her editorship are full of positive news about developing diocesan and parish sacramental programs. Father Richard Hockman CSC began his large output of writings for the Quarterly Publication.

NAMRP members constituted half of the first board of directors of the newly formed National Catholic Office with Persons with Disability (NCPD): Monsignor Thomas Cribbin, Chair, Bishop John Snyder (St. Augustine), Sr. Mary Therese Harrington SH, Brother Joseph Moloney OSF, Mrs. Frances Campbell, and Rev. John Aurelio. New executive director Sr. Rita Baum SSJ, member of NAMRP and the National Catholic Office on the Deaf (NCOD) had previously directed programs for persons with disabilities in the St. Augustine diocese.

In reflecting on his years with NAMRP, Br. Joe Moloney stated, "I have long been convinced that people with disabilities have a diversity of gifts to bring to the community of faith. Church structures that deny or complicate access of people who are handicapped are limiting their own potential of ministry, service, liturgy and understanding of the Word. . . . People who share ministry with people who are retarded find new insights on the Gospel, deeper meaning in fundamental theological truths and a new experience of who God is and how he is present to us."[17]

In an interesting turn, a board president who was not a member of the clergy or a religious order, Ellen Cook, brought in the first parent as executive director, Charles ("Chuck") Luce in 1985. A year later, Sr. Sheila stepped down as editor of *The Quarterly*, making way for a new editor, Marilyn Bishop of the University of Dayton. Prior to her presidency, Ellen Cook had begun a project of stories in *The Quarterly*. Eventually, the stories were published in a book which she edited: *Sharing the Journey, Active Reflections on the Church's Presence with Mentally Retarded Persons* published in 1986 by William C. Brown Company.

During Chuck Luce's tenure as executive director, a project called "On the Move" became a feature of NAMRP activities for over ten years. "On the Move," funded by grant monies, supported consultation services by NAMRP members to give direct aid to dioceses that had not developed any formal programs for persons with mental retardation. These services took many forms and included consultation services, workshops, visits, speakers, and curricula assistance, all directed toward religious education and spiritual formation of persons with mental retardation. There was some attempt to promote their broader inclusion in their faith community. The location of the national office followed the new executive director to Columbia, South Carolina.

One-year terms for officers and annual conferences continued uninterrupted. Membership settled in at approximately 700, generally with the declines in renewals being matched by new members, most often attracted by conference attendance. Conferences, in addition to sharing current concerns and well-known speakers, also developed a social character, particularly among lay members, parents and their children. In addition the Apostolate began closer coordination with AAMD Religion Division, the Association for Retarded Citizens, and NCCC Committee on Disability.

Volunteer editors served the Quarterly and newsletter. Small grants covered publication and mailing expenses. Sr. Ann Vonder Meulen OSF accepted the appointment as newsletter editor in 1986 after Sr. Gabrielle Kowalski OSF became president. The following year Jill Johnson of Cincinnati accepted the editorship of the newsletter. The newsletter began to have more information about Apostolate activities and the concerns of the membership, rather than national disability related items, undoubtedly reflecting the large amount of information now being generated by government, universities and other disability organizations. Newsletters were issued six times a year, rather than monthly.

The Quarterly, under the editorship of Marilyn Bishop, in addition to providing reader friendly layouts, began to raise consciousness about the whole range of abilities within mental retardation, from the medically fragile to those with autism, as well as medical and moral issues. She began to bring an international focus to issues confronting the Catholic Church and its members with intellectual and cognitive disabilities. An educator, she promoted teachers and methods of teaching. She continued as editor until the end of 1993. In that year the Quarterly won an award from the Catholic Press Association for an article by Barbara Stevens entitled "Working in the Community: Opportunities and Challenges: The Parents' Perspective."[18]

During this time, a practice in the bylaws of both the Apostolate and NCPD was to include ex-officio members on each other's board of directors and to participate in each other's conferences and workshops. In 1986, Bishop John J. Snyder, ordinary for the Diocese of St. Augustine, Florida began his 15 years of service to the Apostolate as Episcopal Moderator. A future study was conducted, "Metanoia," to evaluate NAPMR, determining strengths and weaknesses and directions to go. Many interviews were conducted with members and other key persons across the nation. At the 1989 NAMRP conference banquet, Colleen Ruppert, a young woman with Down syndrome, caused a sensation as the featured speaker.

HAPPENINGS IN THE NINETIES AND BEYOND

The decade of the 1990s marked the emergence of for profit providers of services to persons with developmental disabilities. The Americans with Disabilities Act was passed with the hope that the people of the United States would form a more inclusive society. The Catechism of the Catholic Church was published in the United States in 1994, the result of a call from bishops at the 1985 Synod called to celebrate the twentieth anniversary of the closing of the Vatican II Council. While the catechism retained the old order of the Catechism of St. Pius V, the four-part arrangement of creed, liturgy, Christian life and prayer, the material is presented in a new way to respond to the pertinent issues of the day.

In June of 1995, the US bishops issued *Guidelines for the Celebration of Sacraments with Persons with Disabilities*. Paragraph 3 states: "Parish sacramental celebrations should be accessible to persons with disabilities and open to their full, active and conscious participation, according to their capacity."

In 1996, the National Catholic Education Association (NCEA) published a pamphlet entitled "Is there Room for Me," by Sister Antoinette Dudek, Assistant Director of Early Childhood and Special Education Services for the Department of Elementary Schools. In this document, she argued that Catholic schools should promote inclusive classrooms and she held several national meetings entitled, "Making Room for Me." When Sister Dudek left NCEA, unfortunately no successor in interest was appointed.

Pope John Paul II celebrated the millennium with many jubilee days in Rome, including the Jubilee Day of the Communities of the Disabled, December 3, 2000, the day selected by the United Nations for such commemoration. In preparation, the jubilee day committee prepared six theological reflective documents, the chief author of which is Father Enzo Addari. These writings are still available on the Vatican Website.

Scandals involving priests and youth and diocesan neglect erupted in 2002-2003 in the United States. The Bishops continue to address the pastoral and administrative issues raised by these sad happenings.

A study entitled Catholic School Children with Disabilities was published online in 2002 by the Education Department of the US Conference of Catholic Bishops (USCCB). The purpose of the study was to show that the IDEA re-authorization bill should consider the invisible students with disabilities in private schools. The study indicated funding sources for services needed by disabled students in Catholic Schools: IDEA, school tuition, added tuition for services, or other funding. The study did not address those students needing services who were not being served. Seven percent of Catholic school students were identified as having a disability and 1.16 percent of those with disabilities or .08 percent of the total Catholic school population constituted students with mental retardation. Students with mental retardation in Catholic schools slightly outnumbered students with orthopedic disabilities. The USCCB worked with thirteen private school groups to get persons with disabilities in private schools included in the count of students with disabilities as well as to obtain a share of funding for related services for those parents who rejected free and appropriate public education. The lobbying effort resulted in the inclusion of private school students with disabilities in the IDEA reauthorization of 2004.

Anecdotally, the students with mental retardation most likely to enter the Catholic school system are students with Down syndrome. The parents of these students want their children to have an education based on their Catholic heritage. These parents have almost literally pried open the doors of a school for their child and often raise funds themselves for the costs of related services and resource educators.

The United States Conference of Catholic Bishops issued the *National Directory for Catechesis* in the spring of 2005. Subsequent to the 1979 publication of its predecessor, *Sharing the Light of Faith*, the bishops released over a dozen documents, guidelines and letters to address the range of catechesis. The new *Directory* strives to accomplish a great number of issues in a more pastoral manner. For our purposes here, the *Directory* among other things describes the relationship between catechesis and liturgy, provides guidelines for the development of catechetical materials and throughout the document makes specific mention of issues relating to persons with cognitive disabilities and their families.

The Institute of Pastoral Studies at the University of Dayton has supported the Network of Inclusive Catholic Educators (NICE) during this time. NICE held its fifteenth annual conference in 2005.

The President's Committee on Mental Retardation was renamed President's Committee for People with Intellectual Disabilities, by amendment of Presidential Order number 12994 on April 25, 2005 as part of activities surrounding the tenth anniversary of the Americans With Disabilities Act. Although the decision makers felt that the two terms were interchangeable, "intellectual disabilities" was now deemed more acceptable than "mental retardation." In 2004, the committee published "A Road Map for Personal and Economic Freedom for People with Intellectual Disabilities in the 21st Century," available online.

The change of name reflects the current attempt to find a more positive phrase to describe the people among us who learn more slowly and have limitations in judgment and behaviors, including physical abilities, from early childhood. The Association for Retarded Citizens became the Arc and there have been numerous essays on how to address the concerns of self-advocates who have come to feel adversely singled out by the language of the law intended to increase their viability in society. Again, the Apostolate was ahead of the curve when it changed its name in 1997.

CURRENT ERA FOR THE APOSTOLATE

In 1994, Chuck Luce retired as executive director of the Apostolate. The board desired that the national office return to the nation's capital.

The board of directors hired Michela Perrone, who had spent the previous ten years as CEO of the Lt. Joseph P. Kennedy Institute in Washington, DC. At the general membership meeting in Pittsburgh in 1994, a statement opposing the death penalty for person with mental retardation was approved and was subsequently sent to the National Association of State Catholic Conference Directors. The new executive director implemented the substitution of area conferences for one major conference in 1995. A leadership training took place in October of 1995 with twenty participants from fourteen dioceses. Eleven regional conferences were held in 1995. Nevertheless, the Apostolate returned to its tradition and held a national conference the next year.

The board of directors, in a further attempt to generate more excitement sought to develop NAPMR chapters without success. About the same time, NAfIM and NCOD were expelled from their ex-officio posts on the NCPD board. Marilyn Bishop became the staff adjunct for the National Council of Churches of Christ Committee on Disabilities. At the winter board meeting in 1996, Jill Johnson, president, and Bishop John J. Snyder presented a four-pronged approach for accomplishing the mission of the Apostolate: educational, liturgical, social, and service. "Welcome to God's World," a pastoral document developed by the parents committee of the NAPMR board was issued for new parents, hospital chaplains and physicians. Unfortunately, its very expensive format precluded re-publication without a sizeable grant. Ten years later, the Apostolate still receives requests for this brochure.

There was no Quarterly editor when Michela Perrone became executive director. Jill Johnson, president at the time, was also editing the newsletter. Briefly, Robert Dell'Oro acted as editor. Then, Jill Johnson volunteered to supervise all editorial work for both *Quarterly* and newsletter. From then on some, there were some years when only two or three *Quarterly* issues were published.

In 1997, Cheryl Hall of Laurel, Maryland became executive director. All previous executive directors were employed part-time. The new director was hired full-time. However, the Apostolate did not have the income or the ability to generate funding to keep her. She oversaw the thirtieth anniversary celebration of the Apostolate, the installation of a ministry website and the rewriting of the bylaws to allow officers a two-year term. In the spring of 1999, *The Quarterly Publication* produced an issue totally devoted to inclusive Catholic schools. Membership had dwindled to less than 400, and the revenue produced could not support a full-time executive director and the publications. Many priests and religious who had been the worker bees of the Apostolate had left.

Bishops were cutting back on funding offices relating to disability issues.

In 2000, Barbara Lampe was hired part-time as executive director. The volunteer editors had left. At the end of 2001, the last Quarterly Publication was printed. The Apostolate now strives to issue four newsletters a year. Membership has dwindled further. In 2000, 2003, and 2005 there were no conferences. The Apostolate promoted and participated in a pilgrimage to Rome for the Jubilee Day of the Communities of Persons with Disabilities sponsored by the Equal Access Office of the Diocese of Toledo under the leadership of Kitty Kruse.

The Secretariat for Family, Laity, Women and Youth of the United States Conference of Catholic Bishops consulted with the Apostolate and Apostolate members when it produced its online resource *Adults with Cognitive Disabilities/Mental Retardation: Approaches to Adult Faith Formation*. Again, the Apostolate and Apostolate members were asked to critique the first draft of the *National Directory for Catechesis*.

The Apostolate has created a seminary awareness program, produced for the past few years at Mount St. Mary's Seminary in Emmitsburg, Maryland. The website has been greatly expanded.

Here are some of the expected works and dreams in NAfIM's future. Ann Sherzer of the Diocese of Kalamazoo has volunteered to edit an online journal. Kitty Kruse and Grace Harding may be working together on a NAfIM "blog." NAfIM wants to install a curriculum for moral formation on its Website. The Apostolate should articulate important justice issues confronting those of us with intellectual and cognitive differences. There are many social and legal issues. In addition, the Apostolate has been lobbying the U.S. Bishops to be officially concerned about abuse of persons with disabilities including vulnerable adults and to promote the education and "environmental" training needed to bring awareness about this situation. The Apostolate recently passed a resolution to that effect. Improvement in the quality and range of special religious curricular materials is needed. There are two new curricula projects on the horizon, one for children with autism by Cathy Boyle in Massachusetts and one for persons with severe disabilities by Father Bill Gillum OFS Cap at McGuire Memorial in Pennsylvania. Finally, NAfIM expects to enjoy improved relations and collaboration with NCPD, now National Catholic Partnership on Disability, and its current director, Janice L. Benton.

In spite of reduced income and fewer members, pastoral letters and guidelines, the Apostolate remains convinced that the community with and of persons with intellectual, cognitive and developmental disabilities has not lost its need to continue its particular cry within the Catholic Church.

A NOTE ON CATHOLIC SPECIAL RELIGIOUS EDUCATION CURRICULA

In 1984, Dorothy Coughlin of the Diocese of Portland, Oregon wrote the Apostolate about a survey she had made among publishers of Catholic textbooks. She found only one publisher, Winston Press, had addressed special religious education. She proposed that the membership of the Apostolate write to Catholic publishers asking that the situation be corrected.

Most Catholic curricula for religious education intended for persons with mental retardation have the look of the mimeograph or the Xerox about them. Even the well-respected Journey with Jesus series out of Cardinal Stritch University lacks color and gloss. The Gospel Study for that series was first issued in 1978. Even the works of Bridgid O'Donnell, regarded by some as the best and easiest to use, published by Winston Press have a certain black and white quality. There are a number of excellent materials that have also been produced, too many for inclusion in this brief history.

Michela Perrone felt that the situation had to be addressed and she arranged a meeting with Eunice Shriver of the Joseph P. Kennedy Foundation and special religious educators from among the membership of the Apostolate. It was clear to Ms. Perrone that the work involved in creating such a curriculum was not within the resources of the Apostolate. However, two groups from that meeting did make a commitment. One group worked with Grace Harding of the Diocese of Pittsburgh and the other group consisted of Marilyn Bishop and Pat Carter and others at the University of Dayton. Together the two groups produced a two-pronged comprehensive curriculum series and introduced them in 1996.

Although both works together are *The Rose Fitzgerald Kennedy Program to Improve Catholic Religious Education for Children and Adults with Mental Retardation*, the large binder encased developmental Catholic program edited by Grace Harding is the better known work by that title at this time. It is suitable for self-contained settings and an excellent reference for inclusive settings. There are 260 lesson plans and prayer services. A group under the leadership of Mary Brosseau, of the Diocese of Orange, translated the tome into Spanish.

The Dayton program was intended for inclusive settings and provided strategies for adapting existing, mainstream religious curricula and included booklets illustrating these strategies for the Sacraments of Baptism, Confirmation, Eucharist, and Reconciliation. Some publishers of religious textbooks have included these principles in their teaching manuals. The Kennedy Foundation covered the original cost of publishing the materials and for training sessions across the country. *The Quarterly* and the newsletter published training dates for the two programs. The developmental program has sold thousands of copies. Nevertheless, no publisher has published it. Although it is available from Silver, Burdette, and Ginn, the text in a large binder is produced by the Department for Persons with Disabilities of the Diocese of Pittsburgh.

Dorothy Coughlin is still with the Diocese of Portland. If she polled textbook publishers today, she would be hard pressed to find textbooks on religious education for Catholics with mental retardation.

ACKNOWLEDGEMENTS

The Supreme Council of the Knights of Columbus has provided critical and generous annual financial support for the National Apostolate over the years. The author wishes to thank Sister Coletta Dunn, Professor of Special Education at Stritch University for her memories and her encouragement. Discussions with past-president Maryann Rietschlin of Bethpage, New York helped develop the context for writing this history. Past executive director and president Chuck Luce provided written information about his experiences with the Apostolate. Charlotte Shepard kindly spoke to Virginia Kreyer on their behalf about the beginnings of NAfIM involvement with the NCCC Committee on Disabilities. There are so many presidents, board members, episcopal moderators, conference organizers, authors who wrote frequently for *The Quarterly* and newsletter and other members of the Apostolate through the years who deserve a nod for their wonderful presence in this ministry. To you, please accept the authors' apologies that you have not been better served in this brief history. Finally, if a better history is to be told, there should be an emphasis on the spirituality of the many Franciscan priests, brothers and sisters who have journeyed as the Apostolate through the years.

NOTES

1. Pesaniello, Rev. Matthew M., "Why a *National Apostolate for the Mentally Retarded*?" NAMR Quarterly Publication, September, 1968, page 3.

2. Vonder Meulen, OSF, Sister Ann, "A History of the National Apostolate for the Mentally Retarded 1961-1978." 1979 unpublished thesis, Cardinal Stritch University, page 31.

3. Ibid.

4. Wilson, Dolores, "Beginnings Revisited." National Apostolate for Inclusion Ministry Quarterly Publication, Summer 1998, p. 7.

5. Haskett, OSF, Sr. M. Sheila, "The President's View." NAMRP Quarterly Publication, Fall 1978, inside cover.

6. Johnson, Jill, "The President's Message." NAPMR Quarterly Publication, Fall, 1992.

7. "What Is In A Name." National Apostolate for Inclusion Ministry Newsletter, July 1997, Vol. 27, No. 3, p. 5.

8. Miller, Randolph Crump, *The Language Gap and God: Religious Language and Christian Education*, Pilgrim Press, 1970–see Chapter 10 Religion Online prepared by Ted and Winnie Brock.

9. Kieran, Rev. Richard, "Guidelines for the Pastoral Care of the Mentally Retarded." NAMR Quarterly Publication, December 1968, p. 5.

10. Vonder Meulen OSF, Ibid. pp. 11-12.

11. Ibid. p. 7.

12. "Toward a National Catechetical Directory." NAMR Quarterly, Summer 1974, pp. 5-8 and Fall 1974, pp. 16-17.

13. Moloney OSF, Br. Joseph, "Update From the Executive Director." NAMR Quarterly, Special Edition Fall, 1977, p. 3.

14. Foley, OSF Cap, Ed., *Developmental Disabilities and Sacramental Access*, Liturgical Press, 1994, pp. 5-6.

15. Private conversation with consultant Charlotte Shepard, September, 2005.

16. Moloney OSF, Joseph, "Executive Director's Report." NAMRP Quarterly Publication, Fall, 1980, inside front cover.

17. Moloney OSF, Br. Joe, "President's Message." NAMPR Quarterly Publication, Summer 1985, p. 4.

18. NAPMR Quarterly, Summer 1992.

Disability Advocacy
in American Mainline Protestantism

Albert A. Herzog, Jr., PhD, MDiv, MA

SUMMARY. This article provides a brief summary of the disability advocacy in seven American mainline Protestant denominations: the American Baptist Convention; Disciples of Christ; the Episcopal Church; the Evangelical Lutheran Church in American, Presbyterian Church USA; the United Methodist Church; and the United Church of Christ. This history covers the various ministries to the disabled from the pre-1950 era to more recent events including the work of disability advocacy after denominational reorganization. *[Article copies available for a fee from The Haworth Document Delivery Service: 1-800-HAWORTH. E-mail address: <docdelivery@haworthpress.com> Website: <http://www.HaworthPress.com> © 2006 by The Haworth Press, Inc. All rights reserved.]*

KEYWORDS. Disability, disability advocacy, American Mainline Protestantism, ADA, International Year of the Disabled

The ministry of any of the American Mainline Protestant denominations, today, is multidimensional. The simple notion that a religious organization exists to provide for the spiritual needs of its adherents is

---

Albert A. Herzog, Jr. is a Lecturer in Sociology at the Ohio State University, Newark as well as an ordained minister in the United Methodist Church.

[Haworth co-indexing entry note]: "Disability Advocacy in American Mainline Protestantism." Herzog, Albert A. Jr. Co-published simultaneously in *Journal of Religion, Disability & Health* (The Haworth Pastoral Press, an imprint of The Haworth Press, Inc.) Vol. 10, No. 1/2, 2006, pp. 75-92; and: *Disability Advocacy Among Religious Organizations: Histories and Reflections* (ed: Albert A. Herzog, Jr.) The Haworth Pastoral Press, an imprint of The Haworth Press, Inc., 2006, pp. 75-92. Single or multiple copies of this article are available for a fee from The Haworth Document Delivery Service [1-800-HAWORTH, 9:00 a.m. - 5:00 p.m. (EST). E-mail address: docdelivery@haworthpress.com].

Available online at http://www.haworthpress.com/web/JRDH
© 2006 by The Haworth Press, Inc. All rights reserved.
doi:10.1300/J095v10n01_06

immediately made more complex by the realization of the need for such things as a place to meet, worship materials, ministers to lead congregations, and aids to learning the Christian faith. Even more significant (as this paper will show), is that most mainline denominations have evolved numerous organizational structures that provide for a number of ministries which go far beyond the simple and obvious needs of believers who meet together to conduct services and otherwise carry out the "elementary forms of religious life."

EARLY MINISTRIES

Ministries among people with disabilities emerged as a combination of responding to those within a denomination with various impairments needing special approaches and those persons with disabilities on the fringes of society who were viewed as being in need of the ministries of the church. An early example was Ephphatha Missions which emerged from the suggestion of those men who saw a need and related it to the mission of the Norwegian Lutheran Church. They suggested that "the United Church extend its home mission activity to include the deaf and the blind, especially those who belong to the Lutheran Church."[1] A ministry to the deaf and blind was established in Fairbault, Minnesota where a state institute had been established. Out of this effort, a congregation for the deaf was founded as well as several outposts in several Midwestern states.

Within the Methodist tradition, Goodwill Industries was viewed as an early ministry on behalf of people with disabilities. Its leaders and board members were largely ministers in the Methodist Episcopal Church and occasionally in the Methodist Episcopal Church, South. It was started in Boston in 1902 by the Reverend Edgar Helms (1862-1942) as an outgrowth of an institutional church serving inner-city slum residents who had immigrated to America. As Helms led his mission, it became apparent that in addition to a massive program of education and relief there needed to be an effort to provide job skills and experience. The concept and organization of Goodwill Industries grew into a full-scale workshop program to provide the benefactors of the relief effort with a feeling that they had earned the right to purchase clothes and household items. Gradually, the workshop program expanded to include people with disabilities. And, when World War I produced its share of amputees and paralyzed, Goodwill's role expanded to become a leader in the field of rehabilitation.[2]

In the Episcopal Church, ministry among people with disabilities began in 1852 when Thomas Gallaudet was ordained to the priesthood. Gallaudet was called the "missionary to the deaf," and he dedicated his entire ministry to serving deaf people. Gallaudet's mother was deaf, and his father founded the Connecticut School for the Deaf. Gallaudet founded St. Anne's Church for the Deaf in New York City, believed to be the first congregation in any denomination established for deaf people.[3]

Gallaudet was a strong advocate for sign language and played a significant role in the debate between the use of sign language and the widely promoted oral approach. His emphasis on ministry with the deaf led to the ordination of Henry Winter Syles, the first deaf person ordained in any denomination. He and Gallaudet share a feastday, August 27, on the Episcopal calendar of saints.

The Episcopal Conference of the Deaf was established in 1881. Its current president is The Reverend Jay Croft who lives and ministers in Atlanta, Georgia. Today, ministry with people who are deaf is carried out through approximately 70 Episcopal congregations for the deaf. In these congregations, an interpreter is provided for people who visit or are hearing members. In other parishes, a sign-language interpreter is provided for deaf and hard of hearing members or visitors when the majority of the congregation is hearing.

While there is much more that can be written about the early ministries of American Mainline Protestant denominations among people with disabilities, these brief descriptions serve to establish the fact that a strong tradition dates back well before 1950.

WORK OF THE 1950s AND 1960s

A common thread beginning in the 1950s was the ecumenical work of the National Council of Churches which is described in an article earlier in this volume. It can be recalled that many mainline denominations participated in the Council's work with disabilities, especially through its Committee on the Christian Education of Exceptional Persons in cooperation with the Cooperative Publication Association. In addition, each denomination had its own professional staff and publication channels which served the needs of scattered congregations, especially programs focused on the Christian education and camping for persons with mental retardation. These Christian educators saw the need to provide nurture in the faith in a way in which people with disabilities could become full participants in the life of the church. The provision of such resources as curriculum pieces, training manuals, audio-visuals as well as numerous articles in denominational publications combined to provide one base from which Mainline Protestant denominational programs of disability advocacy emerged.

From the late 1950s to the late 1970s, several events took place which gradually pushed mainline denominations away from merely providing services toward advocating for the rights of persons with disabilities to participate fully in the life of the church. In addition to the publication of books, articles and various resources by denominational publishing houses, Mainline Protestant denominations experienced several "grassroots" movements which elevated the needs of people with disabilities onto their national agendas.

In 1960, the General Conference of The Methodist Church, Committee of Hospitals and Homes, acknowledged several petitions expressing concern for the "lack of any Methodist facility to care for physically and [mentally] handicapped children" and called for the Board of Hospital and Homes to "give further consideration to the problem."[4] At the General Conference four years later, the Committee on Hospitals and Homes reported that a study had been conducted and recommended the reading of its report "Methodism Faces the Need of Retarded Children." The Committee also recommended that the General Conference "direct the General Board of Hospitals and Homes to appoint a Committee to seek a cooperative arrangement with one or more Conferences and for Jurisdictions to establish services for mentally retarded children and to promote services to mentally retarded children with a goal of one pilot project by 1968."[5]

At the 1972 General Conference of the United Methodist Church a representative of the Tennessee Annual Conference moved to insert the following paragraph on "Retarded Persons" into the United Methodist Social Principles:

> We recognize the responsibility of the Church to serve and receive the services of retarded persons. Realizing that many of these persons are unable to articulate their own needs and aspirations, we commit ourselves to work with them to articulate and realize these needs and aspirations. We further urge support of programs, services and legislation that will enable them to enjoy their human rights, especially in matters of education, employment, and place of residence.[6]

The title was immediately amended by acceptance to refer to "Retarded and Handicapped."[7] Four years later, the paragraph was further amended in a few small, but significant ways. First, the word "handicapped" was added to the body of the text, rather than as a designation in the title. Second, references to rehabilitation, services, and legislation were added so that the closing sentence read: "We further urge support of programs, of rehabilitation, services, and legislation that will enable them to enjoy their human rights, especially in matters of education, employment, and place of residence."[8]

A similar process occurred among the separate Lutheran denominations which eventually merged to form the Evangelical Lutheran Church in America (ELCA). During the period from 1960 into the early 1970s, national resource services were developed including cassette and Braille access to the Lutheran Standard, Scope, APN Sunday School curriculum, and other print resources of the American Lutheran Church (ALC). In addition, the ALC authorized an "Ephphatha Services Task Force" to explore how its work with the deaf and the blind could serve the entire denomination. It subsequently developed a proposal to expand its services to include those with mental retardation and those with "paralytic and non-paralytic orthopedic disabilities."[9]

Meanwhile, in Lutheran Church in America (LCA), several synods memorialized the national denomination to provide assistance in the form of a staff person and resources for ministry among persons with mental retardation. In 1976, the denomination convened representatives from each of its 31 synods to develop plans for implementing these ministries in their geographical areas.[10]

Another movement that assisted in raising awareness of the needs of people with disabilities on an inter-religious basis was the Healing Community. Founded by the Reverend Harold Wilke, the organization sought to assist congregations in welcoming those who had been alienated by religious groups, including (but not exclusively) people with disabilities. By the late 1970s, the Healing Community had organized several local chapters, published a newsletter "The Caring Congregation," and produced a series of materials for "Access Sunday," materials which are still in wide use today.[11]

DISABILITY RIGHTS TAKES HOLD

The period between the late 1970s and early 1980s were to be the "boom" years for disability rights in American Mainline Protestantism.

The 1976 General Conference of the United Methodist Church referred two petitions expressing concern for the "problems of the handicapped" to its Health and Welfare Division of the General Board of Global Ministries which moved the denomination from providing services to advocacy on behalf of people with disabilities. In 1977, the General Board of Global Ministries authorized the formation of a "task force on ministry to the handicapped and retarded." The following year, an Executive Secretary was hired to staff the newly created Office of Ministries to Persons with Handicapping Conditions.[12] The activities of the Task Force and the opening of the Office of Ministries to Persons with Handicapping Conditions resulted in a significant push to previous legislation and to enact new legislation with regard to people with disabilities and to otherwise set the agenda for the United Methodist Church in the following decade.[13]

In 1977, the 189th General Assembly (1977) of the United Presbyterian Church (U.S.A.) adopted Overture 16 entitled "That All May Enter: Responding to the Concerns of the Handicapped," which called for its "Program Agency to begin exploring possible ministries with the physically, emotionally, and developmentally disabled and to share these ideas with congregations and judicatories."[14] This was followed in 1980 by a consultation on ministries among the disabled sponsored by the Program Agency. Included among the participants were people with blindness, parents of children with disabilities, an adult child of deaf parents, a person with a severe hearing loss, as well as professionals who worked with persons with disabilities, and people with mobility disabilities.

Some of those who had attended the consultation along with others attended the Biennial Conference of the Presbyterian Health, Education, and Welfare Association (PHEWA) held in Louisville, KY, February 5-8, 1981. There, the Presbyterians for Disability Concerns Caucus (PDCC) was formed as a network of PHEWA. The Caucus was organized "to act as a clearinghouse for information concerning disabilities, as well as questions of architecture and attitude; to serve as a place for persons with disabilities to join together to express their concerns and, as a Caucus, to advocate for changing society's (and the church's) approach to disabilities." That these issues needed attention was evident from the many stories members and supporters told about how they were treated by both society and the church. One person told of being asked to get off a plane because her disability was seen as a threat to the safety of the passengers!

In the United Church of Christ, the national program began as a result of grassroots effort.[15] In 1971, its Metropolitan Association of the New York Conference established a Task Force on Exceptional People. This work was largely the ministry of the Reverend Virginia Kreyer. Kreyer had been educated for ministry at New York's Union Theological Seminary and, upon graduating in 1952, was ordained as a minister in the American Baptist Church. For a number of years she retained her ministerial status in an American Baptist congregation in Garden City, New York where she also spent several years working a member of the professional staff of the local affiliate of the United Cerebral Palsy Association. After some time, she left her American Baptist congregation and joined a congregation of the United Church of Christ and still later approached the Metropolitan Association requesting to have her ministerial credentials recognized. The officials were interested but required that Ms. Kreyer have a ministry to which she could be assigned. Subsequently, the Association suggested she assume the responsibility of providing leadership for the Task Force which she was ultimately to initiate and direct.

From 1971 to 1976, the Task Force mounted several efforts to educate congregations in the Metropolitan Association to the needs of people with disabilities. These activities included: giving talks on subjects related to the presence of people with disabilities in society, and in the church; publishing a directory of resources; and encouraging pastors to minister to persons with disabilities and their families. However, the Task Force was not satisfied with the responses to their efforts, and under Reverend Kreyer's direction, raised the question as to whether a statewide and/or national effort would draw more attention to the issues of disability to which congregations would more readily respond.

In 1976, the Task Force decided to present a resolution to the New York Conference. The resolution arrived late and was not considered until its last session. During discussion, a visitor from Japan rose to note that he had traveled across the United States and had not seen one person with a disability. In response, Ms. Kreyer took the floor and gave an impassioned speech in support of the resolution which was then passed unanimously and referred to the next General Synod of the United Church of Christ.

On July 4, 1977, the Eleventh General Synod adopted the resolution entitled "Pronouncement C: The Church and the Handicapped." Both Reverends Kreyer and Wilke gave speeches favoring its adoption. The Pronouncement was prefaced by a "Background Statement" which referred to the U.S. Rehabilitation Act of 1973 which noted that one-tenth of all Americans were "physically and mentally handicapped" and that "most are not seen in church because of attitudinal and architectural barriers." In addition, since most persons with disabilities were "confined" to home rather than institutions, it asked "the United Church to consider their need for participation within the mainstream of community and church life," and called for "special study and action by the congregations, Conferences and the General Synod."[16]

The Pronouncement employed language which, more clearly than other Mainline Protestant denominations, indicated the ties of the United Church of Christ to secular and ecumenical movements for disability advocacy. Its references to recent legislation in the nature of disability rights was in keeping with the denomination's social stance dating back to 1957 when the United Church of Christ acknowledged that it had "faithfully offered prophetic leadership on the major social policy issues of the day."[17] Its Second General Synod in 1959 adopted a comprehensive *Call to Christian Action in Society* which outlined the various settings to which it was called to "pray and work" for "the provision of adequate social services for special groups such as the young, the aging, the handicapped, the mentally ill, and the victims of alcohol and drugs."[18]

The ecumenical nature of the Pronouncement was reflected in the direct quotation of the statement from the World Council of Churches, especially its affirmation "that unity of the family of God is handicapped where these brothers and sisters are treated as objects of condescending charity and derision, and that the unity is broken when they are left out."[19]

Other denominations also responded to the challenges of people with disabilities which appeared in the late 1970s. In 1978, the General Board of the American Baptist Churches called upon American Baptists "to recognize persons with disabilities as integral members of the Christian fellowship and to take immediate affirmative action to enable their full integration in society and in local congregations and in church organizations."[20]

Through the action of the 1982 General Convention of the Episcopal Church, the Presiding Bishop's Taskforce on Accessibility was established. From its inception, the Taskforce was charged with including persons with disabilities into the full life of the church community and with providing resources to meet those needs. It worked to establish a Committee on Disability Concerns in each Episcopal diocese.[21]

IMPLEMENTING DISABILITY RIGHTS

Once the Mainline denominations had passed their respective resolutions through their national legislative bodies, the hard work of implementation began. In some denominations the work was highly
formalized, involving considerable time and money in the form of national committee work and the employment of considerable professional staff time. In other cases, it involved little effort both in terms of
organizational meetings and staff involvement. In either case, the period of the 1980s represented the highpoint of disability rights activism among American Protestant denominations.

With the employment of an Executive Secretary of the Office of
Ministries to Persons with Handicapping Conditions, the United
Methodist Church moved ahead in several arenas. First, the Task
Force on Ministry to the Handicapped and the Mentally Retarded was
organized with representatives from all five jurisdictions (i.e., regions) of the Church which included members with disabilities as well
as professionals with expertise in key areas (e.g., camping ministries
among persons with mentally retardation).

A second thrust was to work toward the enactment of more legislation aimed at adding more weight to previous resolutions. The Task
Force, with the support of its "parent" organization (the Division of
Health and Welfare Ministries), proposed to the 1980 General Conference a resolution entitled "Persons with Handicapping Conditions: To
be part of the whole." In its adopted form, it called "United Methodists
to a new birth of the need to accept, include, receive the gifts of, and respond to the concerns of those persons with mental, physical and/or
psychologically handicapping conditions, including their families."[22]
The resolution listed and briefly described several areas of concern including accessibility, awareness, adequate resources, affirmative action, and advocacy on behalf of persons with handicapping conditions
within the Church as well as in society. More significant, perhaps, was
its successful effort to insert the word "rights" into the United Methodist
Social Principles by asserting that persons with handicapping conditions had the same "humanity and personhood of all individuals as
members of the family of God."

These efforts were also enhanced in rather specific ways such as a
specific change to legislation concerning Diaconal Ministry to state that
"handicapping conditions are not to be construed as unfavorable health
factors when a person is capable of meeting the professional standards
and is physically able to render effective service."[23]

Another approach was to sponsor events and workshops on key issues involving issues of disability and the church. In October, 1981, 34 persons with and without disabilities gathered to explore theological issues related to disability. Several papers were presented, each with two respondents. Later, these were compiled into a booklet titled, "Is Our Theology Disabled?" Two years later, a group of United Methodist clergy and "some ecumenical friends" met to discuss the issue of clergy with disabilities. A summary statement was later released as an "Occasional Paper," by the denomination's General Board of Higher Education and Ministry.[24]

Shortly after the Eleventh General Synod made work among people with disabilities one of "the ten highest priorities of the United Church of Christ," its Executive Council assigned the work to the Division of Health and Welfare which was an organizational arm of its Board of Homeland Ministries. An Advisory Committee was established and soon began its work. The status of the Pronouncement was reviewed and it was quickly decided that "approximately one-half of the committee members should be handicapped and represent several different problems. The other half of the committee should be staff and persons concerned about the handicapped."[25]

Seven objectives were listed which would shape the general goal which was stated as "persons with physical, mental or emotional handicaps and their families will be empowered and fully integrated into the life of the United Church of Christ–and major efforts will be made for their empowerment and integration into society." These objectives, which would shape the denomination's disability advocacy for more than twenty years, were:

1. Develop programs of education and awareness which will sensitize UCC members and society to persons in our congregations and communities who are handicapped physically, mentally, and emotionally.
2. Work toward full integration of handicapped persons and their families into church and society.
3. Removal of physical and architectural barriers which hinder the handicapped from full participation.
4. Training of handicapped through special grants and monitoring of existing government training programs.
5. Work for employer hiring of handicapped persons.
6. Work for changing media images of the handicapped.

7. Maintain an Advisory Committee of the handicapped and others to review the ongoing work of the denomination.

But the stage was not quite set for the Advisor Committee to begin its work. Among other things, there was a struggle with the word "handicapped" which was called into question as referring to a negative stereotype. Reluctantly, the word remained as it was because the "people in the United Church might not be able to make the connection between the committee and the pronouncement."

Also reviewed was the issue of adequate programmatic resources and operating funds for the Advisory Committee. It was stipulated that the Advisory Committee should avail itself to the latest government and secular resources as the basis for an extensive bibliography and that it should avoid "the duplication of efforts," and that it should limit the resources produced by the church which reflected its "unique needs and (our) contribution to the whole area of (the) handicapped."

Funding issues have plagued the disability rights efforts of Mainline Protestants for years, and the United Church of Christ is no exception. Shortly after the Advisory Committee convened, it was estimated that it would cost $21,000 to operate until the next General Synod. A major portion of the needed funds was to be used in support of a consultant (later to be the Reverend Virginia Kreyer) to "work on the coordination of all aspects of the priority," to prepare an educational packet for the Twelfth General Synod, and to provide assistance in arranging three regional meetings on "the problems and issues of the handicapped." In addition, "it was felt that the consultant should be available for speaking engagements around the country." Although these financial issues were never quite settled, enough money was available to carry out the work of the Advisory Committee.

In addition, many tasks were conducted with the assistance of other groups within the denomination and ecumenically. Of the four regional meetings planned, one was held in conjunction with a workshop sponsored by the National Council of Churches and one with the denomination's Protestant Health and Welfare Assembly. Another example was the preparation for the Twelfth General Synod scheduled for 1979. A "hearing" would be held where Harold Wilke (as Chair of the Advisory Committee) would convene and make a brief introduction followed by two presentations–first a theological statement followed by a "handicapped" perspective. A member of the UCC national staff would provide a report on the activities of the priority and Virginia Kreyer presented the Advisory Committee's "future hopes and dreams." Others were recruited to present additional reports and to act as "floor managers" for both the hearings and legislative sessions in which disability issues would be discussed and voted upon.[26]

The legislative action at the Twelfth General Synod resulted in greater clarification of the UCC's tasks with regard to disability issues. It reaffirmed the Pronouncement of the previous General Synod, but directed the denomination's Executive Council to "ensure substantial funding and sufficient staffing . . . for an aggressive and effective approach to the needs of persons with disabilities within the United Church of Christ." In addition, it directed (among other items) "that persons with handicaps be included in affirmative action program within the United Church of Christ," and called upon "Conferences, Associations, and local churches to assess their responsibilities to persons with handicaps and seek ways to eliminate physical and attitudinal barriers which exclude and alienate them."

After the Twelfth General Synod, the Advisory Committee became the UCC National Committee on Persons with Handicaps whose membership eventually represented all areas of the country. A portion of its monies were acquired through a "Neighbors in Need Offering" for "The Handicapped: The Hidden Minority," as well as from other denominational funding sources. Its first actions centered on preparations for the Thirteenth General Synod which would coincide with the 1981 "International Year of the Disabled." These included a special worship service, a booth for display and information, as well as a legislative effort to ensure that meetings at all levels of the denomination would be held in accessible facilities.[27]

One of the "traditions" established by the United Church of Christ (through the suggestion of the Healing Community) was Access Sunday. The denomination's first celebration of Access Sunday was designated for May 4, 1980, but was soon thereafter changed to the second Sunday in October, a date which was already set aside by the United Methodists and the "Lutherans."

The UCC National Committee also had monitored the development of the UCC Affirmative Action Policy. Since the Tenth General Synod voted to establish a policy and to appoint an affirmative action officer, various attempts had been made to include people with disabilities under its umbrella. The 1979 Resolution which affirmed the policy with references to disability resulted in a push by the National Committee under the leadership of its Chair Harold Wilke to "insure Affirmative Action for persons with disabilities and to set up a mechanism for implementation." With the assurance that "extra preferential steps to assure that persons with handicaps will be located, contacted and interviewed," and that an Affirmative Action Statement for Person with Handicaps would be placed in the denomination's *Handbook for Hiring*, the United Church of Christ placed its disability ministry squarely in the arena of civil rights.[28]

Another major event, in which nearly every mainline denomination participated, was the International Year of the Disabled scheduled for 1981. Under the leadership of the National Council of Churches of Christ (NCC) and Harold Wilke and the Healing Community, the United Church of Christ as well as the other denominations worked to highlight the needs of people with disabilities, particularly in relation to their inclusion in the congregation and the larger arenas of denominational life.

The United Methodist Division of Health and Welfare Ministries issued its own pamphlet which described how the International Year fulfilled its emphasis for the 1981-84 Quadrennium, made reference to the actions of the 1980 General Conference, suggested steps congregations could take in response to the presence of persons with disabilities, and provided a list of resources. The General Board of Church and Society's periodical *Engage/Social Action Forum* published a special issue entitled "The Church and Persons with Handicapping Conditions."[29]

ESTABLISHMENT, DECLINE, AND REAFFIRMATION

By the mid-1980s, the American Mainline Protestant denominations had established their respective patterns of disability advocacy. The patterns of the United Methodists, Presbyterians, the Episcopal Church, and the United Church of Christ have been fairly well documented which is not the case for the American Baptists and the Disciples of Christ. All of these Christian communities would experience significant changes in terms of commitment and direction, but "for better or for worse," they developed new ways of disability advocacy in various degrees of continuity with past efforts.

The United Methodists continued to operate with a task force which worked nationally as well as locally in support of disability rights. It called attention to, and revised, periodically, statements pertaining to disability issues in the denomination's *Book of Discipline* and *The Book of Resolutions* which are published after each General Conference. It also worked to support other groups whose issues constitute a part of the disability community within the Church. The United Methodist Congress for the Deaf was organized in 1978 as a "network of pastors who served in deaf ministry and as a way for other deaf Methodists to gather for fellowship and worship"; the Congress evolved into an assembly of representatives from all five jurisdictions with national meetings every two years. After several years, its efforts reached its peak when it (with support of the General Council on Ministries) successfully proposed the establishment and funding of a National Committee on Deaf Ministries. The Committee began its work in 1993 and has made extensive recommendations for various ministries beginning with the 1996 General Conference and each succeeding one in 2000 and in 2004.[30]

A second group which has emerged is the Association of Physically Challenged Ministers (APCM). However, by the time this was organized in 1990, the Task Force had been disbanded and the portfolio of the Executive Secretary had been compressed to become a part of a larger set of duties under the Division of Health and Welfare. A few years later, the Reverend Earl H. Miller was hired as a consultant to guide the program with respect to disability ministry and advocacy. Mr. Miller traveled widely across the denomination and was elected as co-chair along with the Reverend Kathy N. Reeves who was then serving as pastor of a congregation in Chicago. Later, when Miller was killed in an automobile accident, she assumed an executive position on the Division of Health and Welfare, but with a number of portfolios in addition to disability advocacy. Under Reeves' direction, the APCM assumed the position of speaking about disability issues for the United Methodist Church, especially with regard to legislative issues. It continues to operate in various ways, but has not been effective in terms of working with physically challenged ministers as they attempt to pastor local churches. Since the return of Ms. Reeves to the pastorate, the portfolio of disability advocacy has shifted among different staff, although the church has continued to sponsor various committees and advocacy groups, including one focused on the developmentally disabilities.

The National Committee of the United Church of Christ became a mainstay of the denomination as it sought to carry out its work among national service organizations, conferences, associations, and ecumenical groups. As the result of a resolution on mental health which passed the Sixteenth General Synod in 1987, the Committee was actively involved in the founding of Pathways to Promise as an ecumenical substitute for a denominational organization devoted to mental health issues. But by 1992, "it was evident that UCC families affected by mental illness wanted and needed a family voice and presence within" the denomination. As the result, and with the funding of the UCC's American Missionary Association, the Mental Illness Network of the United

Church of Christ began its mission of providing support for families and consumers as well as information and resources for congregational education on mental health issues. The Network interfaces with the National Committee through regular attendance at its meetings and participation in its ongoing work, but has direct contact and involvement with UCC instrumentalities.[31]

However, two events would place the UCC squarely in the disability rights camp. At the meeting of the Twentieth General Synod in 1995, the denomination approved the resolution "Concerning the Church and the Americans With Disabilities Act (ADA) of 1990." Submitted by the United Church Board for Homeland Ministries and the Iowa Conference, it called "on all board, instrumentalities, related bodies, and member congregations of the United Church of Christ to embrace the spirit of the Americans With Disabilities Act (ADA) and hold themselves morally bound by the provisions of this act." The resolution was supported by the National Committee with Harold Wilke speaking in its favor urging its passage "not for the many compelling psychological, social, and economic reasons–there are many–but for the Biblical and theological reasons which compel an affirmative vote."[32]

The second event was the reorganization of the denomination's organizational structure which began in 1995 and extended well beyond the year 2000. As this process was discussed and implemented, the National Committee (now the National Committee on Persons with Disabilities (NCPWD)) sought and obtained assurances that its work would continue after restructuring. However, its eventual placement under what was called Wider Church Ministries (WCM) with its emphasis on health and welfare became a source of concern because its "placement within WCM perpetuates the medical model of looking at disability issues." In addition:

> Persons with disabilities have felt alienated and separated under the medical model. When the medical model is the paradigm, persons with disabilities have been made to feel that their disabilities are what defines them. When that is the paradigm, persons with disabilities, as a group, are "done to and for" and not expected to take charge of their own lives or to contribute to society. The medical model perpetuates the stereotype that persons with disabilities are "*unable*."

In contrast, the NCPWD strongly advocated for a "minority empowerment model," which in their view:

Resulted in the passage of the Americans with Disabilities Act of 1990 (ADA), civil rights law, [that] grants persons with disabilities both dignity and self-determination. This is in contrast to a medical model which emphasizes weakness and dependency.[33]

The NCPWD has repeatedly advocated for coordination of ministries by, for and with persons with disabilities under the Local Church Ministries, recognizing that the most important issue for person with disabilities in the United Church of Christ is full inclusion in all aspects of church life, for both lay and clergy.

In 1994, the Episcopal Taskforce on Accessibility was eliminated when funding for the Office on Social Ministries was reorganized at the national church. Because a member of the Taskforce was unwilling to let disability ministry experience "an unnatural death," she asked if she could be permitted to continue what the Taskforce had begun. Thus, the Episcopal Disability Network was established in Minnesota under the direction of the Rev. Barbara Ramnaraine with funds coming from the national church and donations from individuals and organizations. The Network "serves as a nexus point to inform one diocese about the activities of the others, to provide resources for individuals and congregations in need of such resources, to offer consultative help on accessibility, to maintain a large lending library of taped books about the church and spirituality, and to serve as advocate for persons with disabilities through the writing of resolutions and through addressing discrimination wherever and however it effects persons with disabilities." The Network maintains a Website with links to other organized efforts such as the Episcopal Mental Illness Network, resources, curriculum modifications, and mentoring contacts for people with disabilities.[34]

In the Presbyterian Church, the Presbyterians for Disability Concerns produces the video *Surprising Grace: People, Disabilities, Churches*, introduces persons with disabilities who actively serve their churches, and develops worship aids and a resource packet so that every congregation can celebrate Access Sunday. It has continued to sponsor resolutions before the denomination's General Assembly in order to keep disability issues before the denomination as well as to advocate for disability issues through other church bodies and programs. Through the efforts of members and friends of Presbyterians for Disability Concerns, the Church now has four consultants who are available to the churches and governing bodies of PCUSA. It has also provided "leadership at various conferences on disabilities at Stony Point and Ghost Ranch conference centers and

Resources·General Assembly Committees on Local Arrangements." In 2002, the General Assembly celebrated the twenty-fifth anniversary of the overture "That All May Enter" by making three plenary presentations and having a leadership role in the opening and daily worship services. In 2004, the General Assembly passed a resolution that "all commissioners in future assemblies will have training in disability issues and that the local committees planning the assemblies will also have this training."[35]

The Evangelical Lutheran Church in America (ELCA) currently posts on its website[36] four disability ministries which are anchored historically within its various denominational traditions. The Braille and Tape Ministry "grew out of similar programs of the ELCA's predecessor church bodies," especially Ephphatha Services of The American Lutheran Church which sought to provide for the spiritual and educational needs of its visually impaired members. The Definitely-abled Advisory Committee (DAC) is a sub-committee of the Lutheran Youth Organization Board (BLYO) which seeks to provide opportunities for youth with disabilities experiences in the church and in making their presence known to youth and adults. There is also a "Candle Lighting Service" to highlight the needs of congregants with mental illness and a set of various accessibility resources.

The American Baptist Convention and the Disciples of Christ have continued to provide various disability ministries through benevolent associations, the development of various accessibility resources, and special programs undertaken either by staff with other profiles or by special consultants.

ACKNOWLEDGMENTS

This article is combination of: (1) work of the author on disability advocacy in the United Methodist Church, the United Church of Christ, and the Evangelical Church in America; (2) the contributions of the Reverend Barbara Ramnaraine of The Episcopal Disability Network and the Reverend Nancy Troy of the Presbyterians for Disability Concerns; and (3) additional sources as noted. The author expresses appreciation for these and numerous others who contributed information upon which this article is based.

NOTES

1. Rolfsrud, Erling C. *History of Ephphatha Mission.* Fairbault: Minnesota, Ephphatha Mission, 1959.

2. John Fulton Lewis, *Goodwill: For the Love of People.* Washington, DC: Goodwill Industries of America, Inc., 1977.

3. Information of Episcopal Disability Advocacy supplied by Rev. Barbara Ramnairanie, Personal Communication, August, 2005.

4. *Journal of the General Conference* (1960), 1529-153. (Note: All *Journals of the Genera Conference* are Published by the Methodist/United Methodist Publishing House, Nashville.)

5. *Journal of the General Conference* (1964), 847.

6. *Journal of the General Conference* (1972), 466-467.

7. *Journal of the General Conference* (1972), 467.

8. *Journal of the General Conference* (1976), 1179.

9. "Minutes of the Ephphatha Services Task Force." n.d.

10. Lutheran Church in America, n,d,

11. See Harold H. Wilke. *Angels on My Shoulders and Muses at My Side.* Nashville: Abingdon Press: 1999.

12. Toby Gould. "The Church Needs All its Members," New World Outlook, 36-38, October, 1980.

13. *Journal of the General Conference* (1980), 1332.

14. Information provided by Reverend Nancy Troy. *Presbyterians for Disability Concerns.* 2005.

15. Much of this material is based on the recollections of the Reverend Virginia Kreyer in a telephone conversation with the author on September 2, 1998.

16. *Minutes of the Eleventh General Synod, the United of Christ,* page 53.

17. *The Prophetic Vision: Social Policy Statements United Church of Christ General Synods 1957-1992.* Office of Church in Society, p.v.

18. *Minutes of the Second General Synod,* pp. 171-173.

19. *Minutes of the Eleventh General Synod,* p. 54.

20. American Baptist Association Website www.nbacares.org.

21. See Acknowledgements.

22. *Journal of the General Conference* (1980), 1332.

23. *Journal of the General Conference* (1980), 779, 1214.

24. The United Methodist Center (11/7/83).

25. This information (and following) was obtained from, *Minutes from the Steering Committee Meeting, January 23, 1978.*

26. *Minutes of the United Church of Christ Advisory Committee on Persons with Handicaps, February 22-23, 1980.*

27. *Minutes of the United Church of Christ National Committee on Persons with Disabilities/Handicaps, April 24, 1981.*

28. *Minutes, November 10, 1980.*

29. *E./SA Forum 29,* General Board of Church and Society, no date.

30. See *Daily Christian Advocate, Advanced Edition* (1996), (2000), and (2004). Nashville: The United Methodist Publishing House.

31. Information obtained via internet communication from the Reverend Robert Dell, November 21, 1998.

32. See "NCWPD, Alive and Well at General Synod 22." *That All May Worship and Serve: A Newsletter Of the United Church of Christ National Committee on Persons with Disabilities,* 1, 3 (October, 1999).

33. See "Where Will NCPWD Be in the New UCC Structure?" *That All May Worship and Serve* (June, 1999)

34. The Rev. Barbara Ramnaraine, August, 2005.

35. The Rev. Nancy Troy, 2005.

36. See ELCA.org.

The Christian Reformed Church as a Model for the Inclusion of People with Disabilities

Eric Pridmore, MDiv, MA

SUMMARY. The Christian Reformed Church is presented as a "model" for inclusion of people with disabilities in relation to both society's legislative responses to disability rights culminating in the ADA and the denomination's efforts to include people with disabilities in its religious life. The denomination's decision to "conform" to the ADA is to be located in its theology and its position with respect to social location as an immigrant church with Calvinist leanings. The response of New Hope Church in Atlanta is critiqued as a "test case" of the CRC's ADA policy which indicates mixed compliance. However, the CRC is affirmed as a pattern for other denominations to follow. *[Article copies available for a fee from The Haworth Document Delivery Service: 1-800-HAWORTH. E-mail address: <docdelivery@haworthpress.com> Website: <http://www.HaworthPress.com> © 2006 by The Haworth Press, Inc. All rights reserved.]*

KEYWORDS. Americans With Disabilities Act (ADA), Christian Reformed Church, congregational responses, denominational policies, theology, social location

---

Eric Pridmore is a pastor and college instructor based in Mississippi and is currently working on a PhD in the Sociology of Religion at Drew University.

[Haworth co-indexing entry note]: "The Christian Reformed Church as a Model for the Inclusion of People with Disabilities." Pridmore, Eric. Co-published simultaneously in *Journal of Religion, Disability & Health* (The Haworth Pastoral Press, an imprint of The Haworth Press, Inc.) Vol. 10, No. 1/2, 2006, pp. 93-107; and: *Disability Advocacy Among Religious Organizations: Histories and Reflections* (ed: Albert A. Herzog, Jr.) The Haworth Pastoral Press, an imprint of The Haworth Press, Inc., 2006, pp. 93-107. Single or multiple copies of this article are available for a fee from The Haworth Document Delivery Service [1-800-HAWORTH, 9:00 a.m. - 5:00 p.m. (EST). E-mail address: docdelivery@haworthpress.com].

INTRODUCTION

After several decades of political activism and lobbying, the Americans With Disabilities Act (ADA) was passed into law by the United States Congress in 1990. This act, modeled after the Civil Rights Act of 1964, was designed to challenge the misconceptions, attitudes, isolationist actions, and working conditions that prevent persons with disabilities from gaining access to employment, public buildings, communication services, and transportation services. The ADA made this type of discrimination against disabled individuals equal to discrimination based on a person's race, ethnicity, gender, or religion.[1]

One institution not covered under the provisions of the ADA is the church. During the legislative process church leaders sought exemption from the conditions and regulations of the ADA for two basic reasons: concern by some church leaders over the financial costs of such legislation for small parishes and the belief that there should be a separation between church and state.[2]

This is consistent with the church's history, as over the centuries its response to persons with disabilities has been ambiguous at best. The church has at times posited that disabilities are related to, if not directly caused by, a person's sin. At other times the church has worked diligently to establish agencies, institutions, homes, and resources aimed at ministering to persons with disabling conditions. Overall, however, the church has made little effort to rid itself of the architectural, attitudinal, and communications barriers which prevent people with disabilities from participating in the church. Also, the church has failed to actively invite persons with disabilities into its lay fellowship and professional ministry.

In 1980 the World Council of Churches together with the United Nations announced a special emphasis on the issue of disability. They officially declared 1981 to be the "Year of the Disabled," and throughout the 1980s, the World Council of Churches and most mainline denominations had a strong emphasis on social ministries including ministry with persons with disabilities.[3] However, since the late 1980s these ministries have been of declining importance to the church. According to officials I spoke with from the Episcopal, Evangelical Lutheran Church of America, and the Lutheran-Missouri Synod denominations, financial resources from church members for social ministries (including ministry with people with disabilities) have been shrinking because many members perceive these ministries to be "liberal."

In spite of this lack of interest in people with disabilities shown by most denominations, the Christian Reformed Church (CRC) has shown tremendous leadership and character in complying with the ADA and seeking full inclusion of people with disabilities in all aspects of CRC life. To date, few denominations have made such efforts to be inclusive of disabled persons. As the Committee on Disability Concerns of the CRC has noted, compliance with the ADA is not a matter of conforming to civil law; rather, it is a matter of seeking social justice by extending God's righteousness and justice to all people regardless of their handicapping condition.[4] While the CRC is far from being perfect, its inclusion of disabled individuals can be viewed as a model for religious organizations to follow in its efforts to answer God's call and seek God's justice in this world.

THE NEED FOR JUSTICE

That God's justice is required can be seen from the fact that people with disabilities are among the lowest in terms of economic status of any group in America. The National Health Interview Survey data indicate that people with disabilities are among the poorest of the poor. The likelihood of disability among persons living in the lowest economic levels is nearly double the rate for that of the United States as a whole. The disability rate for households making less than $10,000 is 25 percent. In other words, one in four persons whose family income is $10,000 or less is likely to have a disabling condition which inhibits a major life activity. Moreover, for families with an income of between $10,000 and $19,999 the rate of disability is still a very high 17 percent. A family which is plagued by poverty will probably not be able to provide the necessary familial, technical, or educational resources for a family member with a disability. In addition, a person with a disability living at the lowest levels of the economic system will more than likely experience higher rates of violence, abuse, and abandonment. Impoverished households have few if any resources to deal with the added stressor of a disability.[5]

People with disabilities are among the least educated people in our nation. Thirty-eight percent of those persons with eight years or less of education have a disability while this is the case for only 10 percent of those persons with sixteen or more years of education nationally. Many studies have shown that as the family income level decreases so does the educational level of the family members. Therefore, it is not surprising that people with disabilities are disproportionately represented among both the poorest and least educated segments of our nation.[6]

The relationship of ethnicity to disability marginalizes and hinders the progress of disabled persons even further. Native Americans and African Americans are disproportionately represented among the disabled population. As a result, many persons of color living in the United States are discriminated against and viewed as inferior not only because of their ethnicity but also because of their disabling condition. Native Americans and African Americans are also disproportionately represented among the lowest socio-economic levels. Consequently, persons with a disability in these ethnic groups have almost no opportunity to receive proper training, education, or counseling and are likely to spend their lives living in poverty.[7]

When the ADA was signed into law in 1990, it became the most comprehensive civil rights bill since the Civil Rights Act of 1964. The intention of this Act was to protect people with disabilities from discrimination and unfair treatment as a result of their disability. The ADA is intended not only to protect the civil rights of disabled persons but also to alleviate the economic and educational struggles previously mentioned. However, a 1994 survey commissioned by the National Organization on Disability (NOD) found that little progress had been made in raising the levels of income and social participation among disabled persons. The survey revealed that 68 percent of people with disabilities between the ages of 16 and 64 were unemployed. This survey also revealed that 40 percent of adults with disabilities have a household income of $15,000 or less. In addition, NOD noted that approximately 66 percent of people with disabilities reported that their disability prevented them from becoming involved in community and social activities. To be sure, the ADA is a significant piece of legislation for the disability rights movement; however, this legislation has had only limited success in eliminating the social and economic barriers which hinder people with disabilities.[8]

The Christian Reformed Church is well aware of many of the barriers which impede disabled persons. It is also cognizant of the fact that religious institutions must be a part of the effort to enable people with disabilities to be full participants in society. Since its 1993 decision to comply with the ADA, this denomination has worked assiduously to make all CRC agencies, institutions, and congregations accessible to persons with disabilities–an effort which rests within its rich tradition extending back to the Reformation era in the Netherlands, and its "historic commitment to nondiscrimination, integration, inclusivity."[9] According to the denomination's Committee on Disability Concerns, the denomination as a whole is working to build a community where "people of every race and nation and tongue and ability [are] streaming into the city of God, a new community created from the ruin and misery of humanity."[10]

The CRC is well aware of the need for social justice in religious institutions. It has a long history of involvement in social justice and outreach ministries. This denomination fought hard in the Prohibition movement to maintain restrictions on the consumption of alcohol. It also was integral in establishing Christian labor unions to protect the rights and welfare of workers. During the early 1900s the CRC expressed both sympathy and outrage over the long hours, low wages, hazardous conditions, and the use of child labor. In addition, the CRC has played fundamental role in establishing agencies, homes, and hospitals for the care of people with tuberculosis, the elderly, and persons with mental and physical disabilities. Although theologically conservative, the CRC takes a liberal approach to ministry with and for the poor, oppressed, and marginalized.[11]

Since the 1980s the CRC had become increasingly cognizant of the indispensable gifts and abilities offered by persons with mental and physical disabilities. Moreover, the CRC has become conscious of the sobering reality that many of its churches have barriers that prohibit the disabled from sharing these gifts and abilities. Although secular society has taken the lead in securing the basic human rights of disabled people, the CRC believes that this action by society is "rooted in the heart and intent of God to create a new community in Christ Jesus."[12] Therefore, the denomination maintains that its inclusion of persons with disabilities into the ministry of the church is crucial for the building of God's kingdom. It believes that "the church needs the gifts of persons with disabilities, even as they need the nurture of the church."[13]

Leaders of the CRC contend that though American religious institutions are largely exempt from the ADA, the church's willingness to meet the provisions of the Act should be greater than that of secular institutions. The denominational leaders state that its efforts to comply with the Act are not a matter of complying with civil law, but, rather, a matter of being faithful in ministry. The proposal urging the 1993 Synod of the Christian Reformed Church to vote to comply with the ADA states:

> Moreover, this compliance is in accord with the Biblical charge to share the Good News with all people. The church cannot fulfill its

Biblical mandates without making itself architecturally, intellectually, and programmatically accessible. Moreover, Scripture is replete with examples, concepts, and metaphors that speak to our need to break down barriers and incorporate people with disabilities into the church. To be effective, the church must also find ways in which it can function and have meaning in the lives of people with disabilities.[14]

The ministry of the Christian Reformed Church among persons with disabilities thus illustrates its commitment to following the call of God as well as continuing in the rich religious tradition begun by their ancestors in the Netherlands.

A CRITIQUE OF NEW HOPE CHURCH

For the past twelve years, the Christian Reformed Church of North America has been involved in its process of implementing its 1993 decision to comply with Americans With Disabilities Act (ADA). This process is still unfolding, but it is possible to examine its impact through a study of a congregation in the denomination, New Hope Church located in the Atlanta area.[15] Although New Hope Church is generally not representative of the larger CRC denomination, it is in many ways illustrative of the CRC's commitment to social justice issues. Each week New Hope's worship bulletin usually has a notice telling of the need for mission and ministry in a particular part of the Atlanta area, nation, or world. This congregation also takes up two offerings each Sunday morning during the worship time. The first of these offerings goes to meet the general budget and needs of New Hope congregation. The second offering is a mission offering used to support a selected missionary, congregation, church agency, or some other mission oriented outreach program. There is a different recipient of the mission offering each week. Moreover, I discovered in my interviews that the members of New Hope are very knowledgeable of the different agencies, hospitals, homes, and institutions sponsored by the CRC for those in need of food, education, health care as well as for people with a variety of disabilities. The majority of the people I interviewed believed that the small size and ethnic makeup of the CRC help its members realize the necessity of ministering to the poor and marginalized. As Dutch immigrants many of them know what it is like to be on the periphery of society. New Hope's members exhibit a strong relational connection with CRC members throughout North America and they assert that it is their calling as Christians to minister to each other and to all who bear the image of God.

In my interviews with the members of New Hope I discovered that very few members were fully aware of the 1993 Synod decision to comply with the ADA. Although several members indicated that they had some recollection of this decision, no one could explain how it would impact their own congregation. Despite their lack of knowledge, each member remarked that the CRC's actions were not surprising because it has a rich tradition of involvement with disability ministries and many other kinds of social outreach programs. Although not surprised by the CRC's response to this social justice issue, the action to comply with the ADA has had only a limited affect on New Hope itself. The buildings and facilities of New Hope are quite accessible. A ramp is provided to allow access from the parking lot to the main sidewalk and doors to all three buildings have thresholds which allow for wheelchair access. New Hope also provides accessible bathroom facilities. The worship space is not only well lit but is also on one level, thus providing access to the pulpit and altar area. There are no seating areas in the sanctuary reserved for people in wheelchairs; however, because the pews are moveable, it is easy to make space available to accommodate worshipers using wheelchairs. New Hope is accessible in many ways but it has not done what the Committee on Disability Concerns (CDC) of the CRC has urged all congregations to do.

New Hope's architecture is inadequately accessible in two major ways according to guidelines provided by the CRC. It lacks full access in both the areas of architecture and communications. This congregation has failed to provide handicap parking spaces and designated seating for people in wheelchairs. It has also failed to provide any of the necessary communications resources called for by the CRC. New Hope does not provide hymnals, bulletins, and other worship resources in alternative formats, nor does it provide interpreters or amplification devices for the hearing impaired, nor are videotapes or audio cassettes of church activities provided, and it appears that no educational resources for disabled children and adults is provided. While the members of this church affirm that they are open and comfortable to people with disabilities attending and worshiping at New Hope, they do not give evidence to this in terms of providing the necessary access to full participation for disabled persons. Rather than a proactive attitude about accessibility as recommended by the CRC, this congregation has a reactive attitude. In other words, New Hope will make the necessary changes for persons with disabilities when and if there is a member who has a disability.

There are several possible explanations for New Hope's inaccessibility. One explanation could be the strong congregational perspective. Although the CRC recognizes all legitimate government as being from God and for the good of all society, the attitude of New Hope seems to be that the government of the Synod may be from God but is not necessarily good for all congregations. New Hope Church has reasonably strong connections with the denominational agencies and other CRC congregations; nevertheless, its members put a high value of being an autonomous congregation. The pastor and several members reminded me that regardless of what the Synod decides, it is only a recommendation to local congregations. Although each member I interviewed praised the work of the CRC and the decision to comply with the ADA, they seemed resistant to any requirements by denominational agencies and authorities. This independent attitude is probably intensified as a result of the congregation's distance from other CRC congregations and agencies as well as its autonomy in other ways besides its lack of accessibility. For instance, holy communion within the CRC is typically given only to CRC members and possibly members of other Reformed traditions. However, at New Hope Church, holy communion is offered to all who are Christian and profess Jesus Christ as their Lord and Savior. Also, the worship style of New Hope is dramatically different from other CRC congregations. While this church supports the work of denominational agencies, its primary focus in ministry and service is at the local level. The attitude seems to be that New Hope will become accessible to persons with disabilities when the congregation can discern the value and necessity of doing so.

In his article entitled "Religious Polities as Institutions," Mike McMullen offers a helpful explanation of why the congregational polity of denominations like the CRC would influence how congregations like New Hope Church respond to denominational policy. He notes that a congregational polity is a decentralized form of church government which recognizes the individual congregation as autonomous and authoritative to make its own decisions and govern its own members. The rituals and myths upholding such a polity point to the local congregation as the nucleus of ministry and policy. As a result, it is likely that external motivation will be necessary for a congregation to become aware of denominational policy on a particular issue.[16] For example, New Hope Church, which has a strong congregational ethos, will probably not become fully aware of the CRC's policy regarding compliance with the ADA until a member of New Hope becomes disabled. A church which has an episcopal polity (like the Roman Catholic Church) is able to inform its membership of denominational policy somewhat easier because myths and rituals point to denominational leaders and agencies as authoritative and legitimate.[16]

Another explanation for only partial accessibility at New Hope Church could be the transient nature of its membership. Most of New Hope's members have become part of this congregation as a result of occupational transfers from other parts of the country. Many families are gained and lost by virtue of this transfer process and the membership of New Hope is constantly being reconstituted. Consequently, New Hope lacks the stability and depth found in many other CRC congregations. Therefore, the focus at New Hope is on building a sense of community and unity rather than implementing denominational policies or investing heavily in tangible components. In other words, as a result of constant change New Hope has chosen to concentrate on building relationships rather than accessible architecture and communications. In addition, this transient nature may exacerbate the reactive attitude toward accessibility. For example, New Hope may only choose to pursue greater access for disabled persons after there is evidence that a disabled member will be a regular and faithful member of New Hope. New Hope may not see the value in making extensive changes for a disabled person who may only be a part of the congregation for a short time.

A third reason for New Hope's lack of interest in becoming fully accessible could be its small number of older members. Unlike the typical CRC congregation, a large percentage of New Hope's membership is under the age of 55. Whereas other congregations may fulfill the CDC's accessibility guidelines because there are elderly members who have become disabled as they have gotten older, New Hope is less likely to face this situation. Therefore, New Hope Church will probably not actively pursue full access in all areas recommended by the CDC until a person with a disability joins its membership. This situation may continue to be the case at New Hope until the membership becomes less transient and more stable. Until that occurs, it appears that New Hope Church will continue to maintain a reactive stance toward people with disabilities.[16]

The final and most significant reason for New Hope's lack of access could be related to its understanding of theodicy. The pastor and members I interviewed were reluctant to address the issue of theodicy in any real, concrete way. While they stated that sin does not cause a person to become disabled they also argued that disability as well as all pain and suffering is a result of the Fall. Neither the congregation nor the pastor addressed the issue of why there are people who suffer with disabilities or what role God plays in the lives of those who have a disability. The pastor did state that God had taken on pain and suffering through Christ in order to redeem it. However, this still does not get to the real issue of why pain and disability exist and where God fits within theodicy. It appears that not only is the congregation introverted with respect to its efforts to gain new members but also with respect to issues of suffering and the need for justice. By fully addressing the issue of theodicy the congregation would be more closely connected with the real pain and suffering of people outside the walls of the church. A willingness to discuss this issue would open New Hope to the need for implementing God's justice in this world. Some members of the congregation seemed to dislike the prophetic sermon of their pastor, Rev. Jeon. In fact, Jeon was addressing the need for Christians to recognize the inequity and injustice experienced by many in our nation. Jeon's proclamation that reality stinks probably brought the question of theodicy and the necessity for social justice too near for many at New Hope. The actions to comply with the ADA by the CRC are not merely about meeting particular guidelines and standards. Its compliance also involves the acceptance that justice is necessary for people with disabilities and that this justice will only be gained through vigorous, proactive measures. New Hope is only partially accessible because it has yet to accept the implicit meaning of compliance with the ADA.

THE CRC AS A MODEL

In spite of the fact that the CRC parish surveyed in this paper is only partially accessible, the CRC's actions can be a model for other denominations and religious institutions to follow. One important point which sets this denomination apart is that it is proactive in its approach to ministry for and with people with disabilities. Because religious institutions are largely exempt from the requirements of the ADA, most Christian denominations have done little to incorporate people with disabilities.[17] The CRC has not only attempted to minister to individuals with disabilities but it has also sought to comply with the legal guidelines set for all other societal institutions. The CRC has recognized that many people with disabilities do not attend church activities because they are not able to get to the church, get in the church, get around in the church, or be welcomed by the members of the church. Many people with disabilities have given up attending church because of such barriers while many churches insist that they are not accessible because they have no members who are disabled. The first phase of any denomination's inclusion of persons with disabilities should be that all congregations and parishes are made accessible. And accessibility must go further than ramps, elevators, and special parking spaces. As the CRC has demonstrated, accessibility must be far-reaching and aggressive. Accessibility must include architecture but it must also include making communications, programs, activities, and attitudes accessible. Once inside the confines of the church building, the congregation must enable full participation in worship by making available large print and braille worship materials, proper lighting, hearing devices, designated places for wheelchairs, as well as interpreters for the deaf. In addition, the educational and programmatic areas of the church must also be made accessible. The CRC has shown that Christian education should include special classes for children and adults with disabilities as well as the opportunity to be a part of regular classes. Christian education must also utilize those communications aids and devices listed above in order to make learning accessible in the classroom. However, the most important aspect of access in the local church is the attitude of church members toward the person with a disability. Accessible architecture, communications, and programs will mean little if the person with a disability does not feel welcomed or wanted.[18]

According to the theological and biblical understanding of the CRC, people with disabilities are the image bearers of God. People with disabilities have been created in the image of God and, therefore, must be welcomed into the church and valued as crucial constituents. The church must value people with disabilities as essential to the building of God's new community in Jesus Christ. This new community is one in which people of every race, nation, language, gender, and ability are all welcomed into the family of God. It is not the sin or wrongdoing of a person which has brought their disabling condition. It is not the job of the Church to ensure the salvation of people with disabilities simply because they have a disability. It is the job of the church to welcome and include with joy the image bearers of God who are disabled because they have many gifts, talents, skills, and abilities to contribute to the body of Christ. As the CRC has so eloquently shown, proper architecture and communications are important; however, the accessible congregation begins when the people of that congregation recognize how meaningful people with disabilities are to the life of the Church and, likewise, how meaningful the Church can be for persons who are disabled.[19]

The CRC uses scripture to further define the value of people with disabilities for the Christian community. The CRC has affirmed that in Jesus' ministry people with disabilities were not on the periphery. Jesus crossed many boundaries and broke down many barriers in order to be in ministry with those who had diseases, illnesses, and disabilities. These people had been cast off to the margins of society and were in most cases literally untouchable. Jesus touched them, making them whole in body and spirit. Jesus saw the value of these people. For Jesus, they were not misfits or freaks; rather, they were human beings created by God in love. The CRC has explained to us that scripture is to be the guide for congregations who wish to include persons with disabilities. Those people who would call upon the name of God and yet ignore or inhibit people with disabilities do not know God. Indeed, to really know God, congregations must see all of God's people, including those who have disabilities, as God sees them.[20]

While the CRC's interpretation and application of Jesus' ministry with people with disabilities sets it apart as a model for other denominations, the CRC is also a model by the way in which it provides educational, technical, and financial resources to assist its local congregations in complying with the ADA. The CRC has done more than simply make theological and biblical arguments for the inclusion of disabled individuals. It has gone the next step by providing ecclesiastical support and information. The CRC stated in its proposal to the 1993 Synod that the Committee on Disability Concerns (CDC) will undertake a vigorous campaign to educate the CRC denomination on the issues surrounding ADA compliance.[21] The CDC has gone to great effort to inform people with disabilities as well as CRC agencies and churches of both their rights and responsibilities. Current CRC periodicals and publications have been used to educate members and clarify areas of concern. In addition, the CDC has published a guidebook to disability resources entitled "Opening Doors to All God's People." This book informs local parishes of the rational and basis for complying with the ADA and it gives instructions for doing a self-evaluation of church accessibility.[22] More importantly, this book provides an extensive list of the educational, vocational, government, legal, medical, and ministry resources available to the local congregation. The CRC will also help provide technical assistance to CRC agencies and congregations in the form of architects, lawyers, human resource managers, and others familiar with the ADA.[23] If a congregation finds that it needs assistance in interpreting or implementing the Act, the CDC can help provide resource personnel who can facilitate the congregation's effort to accommodate people with disabilities. As for financial resources, the CRC is cognizant of the fact that many smaller CRC churches will not be fiscally able to accommodate people with disabilities to the extent that larger CRC churches will. Unlike small churches, larger congregations are able to spread the costs of complying with the ADA over a larger membership base. However, the CRC has decided that the smaller congregations are entitled to financial assistance from larger congregations and agencies. Formal guidelines for such assistance have not been delineated but the CRC has stated that financial assistance to small churches is absolutely necessary and will be provided. The Fund for Smaller Churches and the Church Loan Fund are two examples of the fiscal resources which are being made available to smaller CRC congregations seeking to be inclusive of people with disabilities. The CRC intends to make every effort to educate, support, and improve the process of accommodation.

The model established by the CRC is given integrity by the fact that it is a proactive approach to inclusion. The CRC follows the spirit of the ADA by making churches and agencies accessible regardless of whether there are any members or constituents who have a disability. This approach does not force the individual with a disability to accommodate to the church but it allows the church to accommodate and include the disabled community. Most Protestant denominations have developed theological statements regarding people with disabilities and several denominations have agencies which seek to include persons with disabilities. However, most denominations have few rules and guidelines for the inclusion of the disabled community within the local church. Most denominations simply react to individual situations in particular instances. The CRC is a indeed a model for other denominations because it has aggressively sought to include the disabled community rather than waiting for the disabled community to plead for assistance or acknowledgment. The CRC's proactive approach recognizes that the Church needs the gifts and skills offered by people with disabilities and that people with disabilities need the ministry and fellowship of the Church. The proactive nature of the CRC's biblical, theological, and resource-oriented approach to inclusion is the common thread which binds the whole dynamic.

CONCLUSION

While other religious institutions have allowed their exemption from the ADA to generate complacency, the CRC has sought to comply with the letter and the spirit of the Act. Although the CRC's congregational polity may not achieve full compliance within every local CRC church, the denomination as a whole stands as a model for all other religious institutions to follow. The CRC has complied with civil law not because it was compelled to do so, but because it shares the values which undergird the ADA. In his gospel, Matthew recounts that when the Sadducees asked Jesus what the greatest commandment of the Jewish law was Jesus replied that it was to love God with all your Heart, soul, mind, and strength and to love your neighbor as yourself.[24] The CRC's actions demonstrate beautifully its love of God and neighbor. Religious institutions should not be largely exempt from the ADA. But because this is the case it is my hope that the Catholic Church will comprehend the CRC's model for inclusion and respond to God's call for righteousness and justice.

NOTES

1. Along with all other disability laws (e.g., the Federal Rehabilitation Act, the Fair Housing Amendments Act, the Individuals with Disabilities Act, and several other legislative acts) the ADA mandates that businesses, public services, public accommodations, and telecommunications authorities treat persons with disabilities as if their disability was irrelevant and unimportant. A person who is otherwise qualified for services or benefits by the aforementioned entities cannot be discriminated against simply because he or she has a disability. However, the ADA requires not only that a person's disability become irrelevant but also that covered entities "adopt a concept of affirmative action that focuses on the persons' disabilities as well as societal barriers to equal treatment" (Gostin, Lawrence O. and Henry A. Beyer, p. xiii, 1993, "Preface." In L. O. Gostin and H. A. Beyer (Eds.), *Implementing the Americans With Disabilities Act: Rights and Responsibilities of All Americans* (pp. xiii-xvi). Baltimore: Paul H. Brookes Publishing Co.).

2. See *Loving Justice: The ADA and the Religious Community*. 1994. Washington, DC: National Organization on Disability.

3. See other articles in this volume.

4. Christian Reformed Church of North America, 1993, *Opening Doors to All God's People: A Disability–Resource Guide*. Grand Rapids.
Committee on Disability Concerns, Christian Reformed Church of North America, 1993, *Toward Full Compliance with the Provisions of the Americans With Disabilities Act in the Christian Reformed Church of North America: A Report to Synod 1993*. Grand Rapids.

5. Inez Fitzgerald Storck and Susan Thompson-Hoffman, 1991, "Demographic Characteristics of the Disabled Population." In I. F. Storck and S. Thompson-Hoffman (eds.), *Disability in the +United States: A Portrait From National Data* (pp. 15-33). New York: Springer Publishing.

6. Ibid.

7. Ibid.

8. N.O.D./Harris Survey of Americans with Disabilities (pp. 10-20) New York: Harris and Associates, 1994.

9. Committee on Disability Concerns, Christian Reformed Church of North America, 1993, *Toward Full Compliance with the Provisions of the Americans With Disabilities Act in the Christian Reformed Church of North America: A Report to Synod 1993.* Grand Rapids. p. 7

10. Ibid., p. 3.

11. James D. Bratt, 1984, *Dutch Calvinism in Modern America: A History of A Conservative Subculture.* Grand Rapids: Wm. B. Eerdmans.

12. Committee on Disability Concerns, Christian Reformed Church of North America, 1993, *Toward Full Compliance with the Provisions of the Americans With Disabilities Act in the Christian Reformed Church of North America: A Report to Synod 1993.* Grand Rapids. p. 7.

13. Ibid.

14. Ibid., p. 8.

15. This study was conducted as part of an M.Div. Honors thesis at Candler School of Theology at Emory University in Atlanta, Georgia. The study was conducted during the fall of 1995 and the spring of 1996.

16. McMullen, John Michael, 1994, "Religious Polities as Institutions." *Social Forces.* 27 (2): 709-728.

17. I am not aware of any feedback on the issue of size which has been reported in CRC publications.

18. I make this assertion based, in part, on the NOD survey results that indicate that persons with disabilities are much less likely to be involved in religious and community activities than non-disabled persons even though the disabled indicated a greater interest in attending such activities than did the non-disabled respondents. In addition, I have come to this conclusion after reviewing the policy statements of the five largest Christian denominations. See also: Janet Miller Rife and Ginny Thornburgh, 1996, *From Barriers to Bridges: A Community Action Guide for Congregations and People with Disabilities.* National Organization on Disability.

19. Janet Miller Rife and Ginny Thornburgh, 1996, *From Barriers to Bridges: A Community Action Guide for Congregations and People with Disabilities.* National Organization on Disability.

20. Committee on Disability Concerns, The Christian Reformed Church of North America, 1993, *Toward Full Compliance with the Provisions of the Americans with Disabilities Act in the Christian Reformed Church of North America: A Report to Synod 1993.* Grand Rapids.

21. Ibid.

22. Committee on Disability Concerns, The Christian Reformed Church of North America, 1993, *Opening Doors to All God's People: A Disability–Resource Guide.* Grand Rapids.

23. Ibid.

24. Mark 12:33

The Religion and Spirituality Division
of the American Association
on Mental Retardation

Dennis Schurter, DMin, MDiv

SUMMARY. The author summarizes the beginnings of the AAMR Religion and Spirituality Division from 1960-1983. He then describes in more detail the growth of the organization in the 1980s and 1990s. Three broad areas of the Division's activities are discussed: (1) interfaith dialogue and interdisciplinary collaboration; (2) the development of resources to support the practice of religion and the spirituality of persons with intellectual disabilities; and (3) efforts to support professionals in ministry with people with disabilities. Future directions of the Division are summarized. *[Article copies available for a fee from The Haworth Document Delivery Service: 1-800-HAWORTH. E-mail address: <docdelivery@ haworthpress.com> Website: <http://www.HaworthPress.com> © 2006 by The Haworth Press, Inc. All rights reserved.]*

KEYWORDS. History, religion, spirituality, disabilities, interfaith, resources

---

Dennis Schurter recently retired after thirty years as Chaplain at Denton State School in Denton, TX.

[Haworth co-indexing entry note]: "The Religion and Spirituality Division of the American Association on Mental Retardation." Schurter, Dennis. Co-published simultaneously in *Journal of Religion, Disability & Health* (The Haworth Pastoral Press, an imprint of The Haworth Press, Inc.) Vol. 10, No. 1/2, 2006, pp. 109-126; and: *Disability Advocacy Among Religious Organizations: Histories and Reflections* (ed: Albert A. Herzog, Jr.) The Haworth Pastoral Press, an imprint of The Haworth Press, Inc., 2006, pp. 109-126. Single or multiple copies of this article are available for a fee from The Haworth Document Delivery Service [1-800-HAWORTH, 9:00 a.m. - 5:00 p.m. (EST). E-mail address: docdelivery@haworthpress.com].

Available online at http://www.haworthpress.com/web/JRDH
© 2006 by The Haworth Press, Inc. All rights reserved.
doi:10.1300/J095v10n01_08

The Religion and Spirituality Division of the American Association on Mental Retardation (AAMR) differs in some respects from free-standing organizations. The primary difference lies in the fact that the Division is part of a larger professional association. It is one of sixteen divisions and ten "special interest groups" (SIGs) representing various professional disciplines in the field of developmental disabilities.[1] The Religion and Spirituality Division has approximately 170 members participating within the 5,500-member AAMR. On the one hand, this organizational structure has established limits to the Division's ability to participate in some cooperative activities with other organizations. For example, the Division has not been able to function fully within the Coalition on Ministry in Specialized Settings (COMISS) because of financial limitations. On the other hand, being part of a larger professional interdisciplinary organization has created opportunities for dialogue and collaboration with professionals in many other areas who are also concerned about improving the lives of people with disabilities. Many other examples will illustrate this as we pursue the story of the Religion and Spirituality Division.

THE DIVISION'S EARLY HISTORY[2]

The Religion and Spirituality Division was born in 1960. Don Lawson, appointed chaplain at the Caswell Center in North Carolina in 1958, presented a paper at an Education Division session in the 1960 AAMD meeting in Baltimore.[3] His paper was titled, "A Survey of Present Trends in Religious Education of Mentally Retarded Persons in State Institutions." Three other chaplains approached Lawson after his presentation, and together they decided to organize a network of chaplains and other religious workers within the AAMD. In 1965 their efforts bore fruit as the national organization recognized the "Sub-section for Chaplains and other Religious Workers" as part of the Administration Division.

This core group of Protestant chaplains included Don Lawson, Howard Parshall, Vincent Mostrom, Bert Streufert, and Herbert Graening. They soon attracted Catholic chaplains George Kuryvial, Charles Bauer, and Ralph Karl. Together they intentionally recruited members from other divisions and disciplines.

The momentum continued, and in 1968 the name of the sub-section was changed to the "Religion Sub-section," intentionally reflecting the fact that chaplaincy was not the only form of ministry with people with developmental disabilities. Marshall Nelson from the Lutheran Church–Missouri Synod and Ima Jean Kidd, on the staff at the National Council of Churches, became the first non-chaplain officers in the sub-section.

In 1971 there were two pivotal developments for the organization and its members. First, after eleven years of sharing a short, quarterly newsletter, the Sub-division gave birth to *Information Service*, a quarterly newsletter/journal, edited by Father Ralph Karl, then president of the Sub-division. In 1974 Reuben Johnson, chaplain at Gracewood State School in Georgia, became the editor. This publication would provide a greater voice for faith concerns within the AAMD and become an avenue for sharing among ministry professionals in the field.

Second, the Sub-division had discussed certification and accreditation issues for five years. In 1971 it supported the formation of the Religious Certification Agency for Retardation (RCAR), a separate incorporated body organized in conjunction with the Committee on Religious Nurture of the Association for Retarded Children. The RCAR would encourage professional religious workers to recognize the value of their ministries and to claim the competence to provide leadership in matters of faith. Meanwhile, the Sub-division was growing as membership reached 125.

In 1977 Don Lawson completed his second term as chair of the Sub-division and presided over the celebration of the group's achieving "Division" status. When the Sub-division passed the 200-member milestone, the AAMD granted it the status of Religion Division. At that year's convention in New Orleans, Sister Mary Sullivan from Rhode Island became the first woman to be vice-president (or chair) of the Division. Membership continued to climb to nearly 300 in 1979.

"Then, in 1979, a number of changes led to a five-year decline in membership. Many of the original leaders reached retirement age. *Information Service* was cut back because of funding changes for AAMD divisions and suspended in the early 1980s when Reuben Johnson retired. RCAR lost many of its leaders to retirement, but more importantly its certification was not required by any hiring or accrediting agency. More and more people were entering the field of ministries with persons with developmental disabilities, but other national networks, primarily connected to faith groups, were growing, including the National Apostolate with Mentally Retarded Persons, the National Catholic Office for Persons with Disabilities, the Healing Community, and denominational advocacy and resource networks" (Gaventa, p. 268). The Division was entering a time of decline and approaching an opportunity for redefinition.

OPPORTUNITY FOR RENEWAL

At the 1983 AAMD national convention in Dallas, Texas, the Religion Division found itself in a disorganized state. Few members were in attendance. Division program sessions were not well promoted or attended. There did not seem to be a cohesive leadership within the Division. That year in Dallas, Bill Gaventa was installed as the newly-elected president of the Division. In 1984 he proposed a series of steps to improve continuity of leadership and to stimulate a sense of vision within the Division. He proposed (1) the development of "formal interest groups" within the Division, e.g., institutional ministries, religious education, residential ministries, etc.; (2) the development of a certification committee for ordained and lay ministries; (3) the establishment of an executive secretary "to meet the primary need of providing more continuity and sharing in leadership with the President"; (4) the establishment of a publication committee; and (5) the establishment of an executive committee for the Division.[4] While these five proposals have evolved in various ways, these ideas have formed the core of the vision that has shaped the Division's identity and mission in the years since 1983.

To pursue this development, we will look at the history of the Division's organization and structure following Gaventa's 1984 proposal. We will then look at its history in three areas: (1) the Division as an arena for interfaith dialogue and as a bridge for collaboration with so-called secular professionals and services both inside and outside the AAMR; (2) the Division's efforts to share resources and promote a growing literature in the field of spirituality and disabilities; and (3) its efforts to support and empower religion professionals in their diverse ministries with and for people with developmental disabilities.

A MATURING ORGANIZATION

Following on Gaventa's proposal, the Division in its 1985 meeting in Philadelphia voted to establish an executive committee with officers serving four-year terms. The president of the Division would still be elected through the AAMD national election process for a two-year term. Executive committee members in 1985 included Bill Gaventa as executive secretary, Glenn Henricksen as publications committee chair, and John Hedrick as recording secretary and treasurer.

This executive committee structure allowed the Division to elect a stable leadership who would provide consistency to the Division's programs and vision even as the biennial election of a new president followed the guidelines of the national organization. In 1991 Division members were asked to evaluate the position of executive secretary, and in the meeting in Arlington, Virginia, they asked Gaventa to continue in that position for two years. In 1993 in Washington, D.C., the membership asked him to serve another five year term in this volunteer position. At that time members also urged the development of by-laws and a more elaborate organizational structure to guide the Division.

In 1996 with the guidance of immediate past-president Brett Webb-Mitchell, the Division approved "A Covenant: The By-Laws of the AAMR-Religion Division." This document described the election and duties of the Division president, past-president, executive secretary, treasurer, newsletter editor, book exhibit coordinator, and the structure of the Certification Committee. With revisions and amendments the following year, the Covenant has been the guiding document for the governance of the Division. The challenge continues to be finding volunteer leadership to fill the positions.

When the need for a mission statement was raised, a trio from Chicago came forward to prepare a draft. Julie Hess, Elizabeth Sivek, and Jeanne Valenti presented a first draft in the 1989 AAMR meeting in Chicago. The final revision of the mission statement was approved in 1991 in the Arlington meeting as follows.

Preamble

The Religion and Spirituality Division of the American Association on Mental Retardation is an interfaith, interdisciplinary association of professional, ordained, and lay people who journey with persons with developmental disabilities and with their families.

Mission Statement

Our mission is to share resources which foster opportunities for spiritual growth for persons with developmental disabilities while respecting their religious identity.

Goals

1. To foster inclusion of persons with developmental disabilities and the sharing of their gifts and graces in the total life of the congregation and the community.

2. To provide a forum for dialogue to creatively foster religious education programs that are life-long and age appropriate.
3. To work cooperatively with all divisions of AAMR to enhance the spiritual supports available to persons with developmental disabilities and to their families.

The first mention of suggestions to change the name of the Division appeared in the winter, 1995, edition of the quarterly newsletter. After several years of discussion concerning the name of the Division, the members in the 1999 business meeting decided to seek input from the membership through a survey in the newsletter. The survey requested attitudes and comments concerning changing the name to the Religion and Spirituality Division. The idea of including "spirituality" in the name of the Division was prompted by several factors: (1) emphasis in the literature on spiritual supports for people with developmental disabilities and the recognition of the spiritual nature of all people; (2) spirituality is a broader concept than religion and religious practice; and (3) the idea of addressing the spiritual issues, gifts, and needs of people with disabilities was a more adequate expression of the mission of the Division than simply using the concept of religion.

In the June, 2000, business meeting the Division voted to proceed with a ballot on a name change, asking members to approve the name "Religion and Spirituality Division." The ballot was included in the October voting for national and division officers. The name change was approved and officially sanctioned by the AAMR board following the election.

While the organizational structure of the Religion and Spirituality Division has evolved over the past twenty years, it has only been the handmaid of the Division as it has sought to fulfill its vision in three other areas. Thus, we turn to these three.

A VISION OF DIALOGUE AND COLLABORATION

Interfaith dialogue and interdisciplinary collaboration had been goals of the Religion and Spirituality Division since its inception in 1960. Following the 1983 AAMD national conference in Dallas, these goals needed to be addressed in fresh ways. The Division leadership focused on several concerns, including mainstreaming the Division into the AAMD, interfaith dialogue within the Division, interdisciplinary participation in AAMD programs, and ways the Division could bring faith and spirituality concerns to bear within the AAMD as on organization.

To make a beginning, the Division requested that the 1984 national conference program include interfaith sessions for meditation and reflection each morning. These half-hour sessions, led by members of the Division, provided opportunity for all AAMD members to gather for a time of interfaith reflection/prayer/meditation at the beginning of each day. The sessions also aimed to show the diversity of spiritual expressions inherent in peoples of all faiths, those with and without obvious disabilities.

Through the past twenty years these sessions for reflection have frequently been quiet opportunities for sharing, story telling, sacred readings, and prayer. At other times, they have been lively expressions of the diversity of spirituality in our American culture. The three morning sessions in the 1987 conference in Los Angeles featured the "High Hopes" vocal group, Jewish dances led by a rabbi, and the film "Blessed Be." In San Diego in 1998 the morning meditations included Native American dances, Jewish mysticism, and an African American choir. In that year Stanley Herr, then president of the AAMR, stopped by to share the morning session and was enthralled by the Native American dancers in full regalia. He invited the dance troupe to perform at the opening plenary session that morning, and they were welcomed with enthusiasm from the entire conference.

Division members also participated in more academic approaches to integrating spirituality and faith concerns into the life and thinking of the AAMR organization. In the 1991 conference in Arlington, AAMR leaders presented a draft of the 1992 edition of *Mental Retardation: Definition, Classifications, and Systems of Support.* Chapter 9 was written by Dr. Robert Schalock and titled "Appropriate Supports." This chapter contained the first discussion in an AAMR publication of spirituality and spiritual supports through faith communities. Members of the Division promoted the inclusion of spirituality issues in this publication, but a key factor was the fact that Dr. David Coulter, a Division member, was also on the publication committee for the book. After the book's publication, the Division planned its "retreat" at the 1996 conference as a half-day symposium on spirituality and the definition of mental retardation. The key speaker was Dr. David Coulter with responses and presentations from others in the Division.

In another successful effort, Division members Roger Peters and Bill Gaventa participated in development of the AAMR "Statement on Spirituality and Religious Freedom" in 2001. This was later revised and accepted as a joint statement of the AAMR and The Arc in 2002.

Along with its concern with integrating spirituality and faith issues into the larger AAMR organization, the Division sought to create a spirit of collaboration between the Religion and Spirituality Division and the other professional disciplines within AAMR. Given the Division members' wholistic understanding of human nature, they recognized that every other discipline had something to contribute to the dialogue concerning human services. The Division's goal was to listen as well as to speak to others.

Multidisciplinary program sessions at national conferences offered excellent opportunities for this kind of dialogue and collaboration. Division members actively sought to create such sessions in the conference programs. One example of the multidisciplinary programs at annual conferences was noted in the "1992 Religion Division Report to the AAMR Board of Directors": "Division presentations on family supports, genetics, socio-sexuality education, ethics, religious education and worship, and ADA were well attended. Several Division members gave a presentation on religious services to the Community Division."

At the 1991 conference in Arlington, Virginia, the Division conducted a symposium titled "The ADA: A Mandate for Creating Caring Congregations." Participating in the symposium were representatives from the U.S. Attorney General's office, the National Organization on Disabilities, Focus, Inc., the National Catholic Office on Persons with Disabilities, the Board of Jewish Education of Greater Washington, and Joni and Friends.[5] In the Denver conference in 2001, the Division planned collaborative sessions with the Creative Arts Therapy Special Interest Group[6] and the Medicine and Nursing Divisions. Such national conference sessions created opportunities for dialogue and friendships within a diverse interdisciplinary environment.

Interfaith dialogue and networking among religious professionals was another goal of the Division. Catholics and Protestants, institutional and community workers had been a part of the Division membership since its beginning. In 1991 there were increased efforts to broaden the AAMR base in the Jewish community with several new members joining in that year. Jewish members were also encouraged to participate in conference lecture and poster sessions and to lead morning meditation sessions.

International networking also grew in the 1990s. During these years new members joined the Division from Israel, the Bahamas, Germany, Taiwan, Canada, England, Singapore, and Australia. David Hughes from the United Kingdom presented a paper at the 1994 conference and later contributed articles to the Division newsletter. The International Association for the Scientific Study of Intellectual Disabilities (IASSID) held its 2000 conference in Seattle. Division members David Coulter and Bill Gaventa organized a series of conference sessions on the theme of spirituality and health. This was the first time spirituality issues had been addressed in this organization. Other Division members attended the conference. Through an e-mail contact with an individual in Czechoslovakia, the Division sent resources and materials to an organization serving people with disabilities in that country.

Two other strategies have been important to the vitality of the Division and its internal networking–the annual retreats and the Division dinners. Both have taken place at annual conferences and have played vital roles in building friendships among members and encouraging new members to join. Annual retreats have been half to full-day events just preceding the opening of the national meeting. They have included a wide variety of programs and speakers, including Stanley Hauerwas (1986), Howard Clinebell (1987), and Sister Sue Mosteller (2001). The 1990 retreat in Atlanta included a march to the Martin Luther King memorial and speech by Coretta King. In Washington, D.C., in 2000 the group gathered at the Art and Drama Therapy Institute, which provides day programs for adults with developmental disabilities.

Division dinners have been a social highlight of the conferences with as many as one hundred people in attendance in 1987. In these events friendships are made and nurtured as members of the Division become reacquainted and some from other divisions join the festivities. The venues have included the Potter's House in Washington, D.C. (1993), Chinatown in San Francisco (1995), the "floating banquet tables" on the San Antonio River (1996), and a Greek restaurant in New York City (1997) following a tour of the Cathedral of St. John the Divine.

A final aspect of the Division's collaborative efforts is its activities to reach beyond the AAMR to other organizations. Chief among these has been its participation in the Coalition on Ministry in Specialized Settings (COMISS), more recently known as the Network. The Division became involved in the COMISS network in 1984 through the efforts of then-president Bill Gaventa. In 1985 Gaventa and Division president Nancy Lane attended the COMISS meeting. In 1988 Division members participated in Dialogue '88, a major national conference involving many national organizations involved in spiritual care. Dialogue '94 was the next COMISS conference in Milwaukee, and the Division co-sponsored two activities with other disability-related organizations–a breakfast event and a workshop led by John McKnight. The Division's resource exhibit was on display, and several Division members led a workshop on congregation advocacy.

The Division has continued through the years to participate in COMISS activities to the extent possible. In 1997 Roger Peters began attending COMISS meetings as the primary Division representative. Other COMISS members have welcomed the Religion and Spirituality Division, but circumstances have hampered full participation. As part of a larger interdisciplinary organization, the Division has lacked the freedom to operate as an independent entity and has not had the financial resources to participate fully in COMISS task force projects and meetings. The Division's participation has always depended on the individual members who were willing to attend COMISS meetings. Nevertheless, the efforts have been worthwhile because of the opportunities to network with other ministry organizations and to share concerns and raise awareness about ministry with people with disabilities of all kinds.

Other collaborative efforts have included cooperation with *Exceptional Parent* magazine in publishing an issue on religious education (1994), contributing $1,500 to Robert Perske's effort to produce a video on death row inmate Johnny Lee Wilson (1995),[7] and becoming a sponsor of the Accessible Congregations Campaign of the National Organization on Disabilities (NOD) (1998). The Division has joined in other cooperative projects with the National Apostolate for Inclusion Ministry (NAfIM), the National Council of Churches Taskforce on Disabilities, the National Catholic Office on Persons with Disabilities, the Arizona Council for Jews with Special Needs, the Arc, and the Religion and Disabilities Program of the NOD.

TOWARD A LARGER BODY OF KNOWLEDGE

Throughout its 128-year history the AAMR has sought through its national organization and its various divisions to advance research in the field of cognitive disabilities and to inspire the best practices for providing services to those in need of such services. The Religion and Spirituality Division has pursued this same objective by organizing and promoting information concerning resources in the fields of religious practices, spiritual supports, and community integration. Division leaders have striven to increase the body of literature in this field in order to support persons with cognitive impairments and their families, religion professionals in all areas of ministry, and agencies and congregations seeking to serve those with disabilities. Through the years the Division has used various strategies to meet these objectives, including the Division newsletter, the Cooperative Resource Exhibit, and the development of various publications.

The Division newsletter began in the 1960s as an effort to build the network of the "Sub-section of Chaplains and Other Religious Workers." Periodic mailings strove to keep the group members informed of conference plans and to share resources. The newsletter waned in the late 1970s until 1983 when it was revived with the purposes of sharing information about Division activities, creating a network among members, and sharing resources for ministry. In 1988 Bethesda Lutheran Homes and Services of Watertown, Wisconsin, began printing and mailing the quarterly publication. In 1991 the Division began offering the newsletter to non-members as a two-year subscription for $10 in order the share resources and encourage membership in AAMR. Currently, the subscription rate is $25 for three years for non-members.

In 1993 there was an expansion of the newsletter to include articles related to other agencies that shared the Division's vision for ministry. They revealed a growing cooperation with other groups. In addition, Division members were asked to help compile a mailing of list of seminary representatives, "people who would help share ideas about new resources, give us news about writings or resources related to people with disabilities, and be contacts for students who are doing work in this area of ministry" (Division newsletter, spring, '94). The fall issue in 1994 had the first article for the "Seminary Education Column" edited by Marilyn Bishop and later by Peggy Dunn. The summer issue of that year included the first entry for the "Jewish Perspective Column" written by Becca Hornstein, who continues to edit the column. The spring issue in 1999 had the first article contributed by an overseas member, David Hughes from the United Kingdom.

In 1999 the executive secretary's annual report to the Division stated that 500 copies of the newsletter were distributed with about 250 copies going to Division members. Others were mailed to the AAMR leadership, seminary professors, COMISS members and leaders, paid subscribers, and complementary copies. This small, quarterly publication (usually 8-12 pages) continues to be a mainstay for its readership as it shares resources, best practices, and information about the activities of the Division and other organizations.

The Cooperative Resource Exhibit was first assembled in 1984 at the national conference in Minneapolis. Publishers and resource suppliers were given opportunity to send single copies of books and other resources for display in the exhibit for a rate of $25 per entry. Areas of interest included in the exhibit were theology and religion resources, education curricula for congregational awareness and religious education for people with developmental disabilities, community-building resources, and inspirational books, videos, etc. In 1992 the exhibit included resources from 49 suppliers. The exhibit continues to be a popular display at AAMR national conferences, but it has also visited many other national and regional meetings of various disability and ministry organizations.

The third direction in expanding the body of knowledge concerning spiritual and ministry resources has been the Division's efforts to promote publications in the form of journals. First steps were taken in 1971 when the Division began *Information Service*, edited by Father Ralph Karl. This quarterly newsletter/journal published papers from conference presentations as well as Division news. It was discontinued in 1983, and in 1985 the first issue of *Occasional Journal of Religion and Developmental Disabilities* was published with the Division papers from the 1984 conference. The *Occasional Journal* was edited by Glenn Hendricksen for two years and later by Ingram Parmley. The last issue was published in 1991 with Division papers from the 1989 AAMR conference.

In the meantime, Parmley was also coordinating initial planning for a journal of religion and developmental disabilities to be published professionally. In 1988 the AAMR board of directors approved plans for a *Journal of Religion and Developmental Disabilities* under the editorship of Louis Heifitz. Various negotiations continued for three years until in 1991 agreement was reached with The Haworth Press, Inc. for the publication of the *Journal of Religion in Disability & Rehabilitation*, edited by William Blair and Dana Davidson. The quarterly journal under this title produced two volumes in 1994-1996. With the declining health of the editors, the journal ceased publication.

In the winter of 1999 the Division newsletter announced that the journal would be revived as the *Journal of Religion, Disability, & Health (JRDH)* with David Coulter and Bill Gaventa as co-editors. Both were members of the Division, and the journal proceeded with the support of the Division. Vol. 3, No. 1 included material organized by the previous editors. Issue No. 2 was published under the guidance of Coulter and Gaventa.

Special issues of the *JRDH* have included collected papers from the IASSID conference in Seattle in 2000 (Vol. 5, No. 2-3), selected writings of Wolf Wolfensberger (Vol. 4, No. 2-3), pastoral writings of Robert Perske (Vol. 7, No. 1-2), and collected articles on disability and spirituality from Australia (Vol. 8, No. 1-2). Some of these special issues have been republished as separate books by The Haworth Press, Inc.

In 2000 the Division completed an "affiliation agreement" with Haworth Press through which they shared advertising benefits and the Division members received reduced subscription rates for the *JRDH*. While the journal is not strictly speaking a product of the Division, support from Division members and editorship by Division leaders have made the *JRDH* possible. The journal continues to contribute to the body of knowledge in the field of spirituality and disability and to encourage others to write and to further research and practice in the field.

One final contribution from the Division is the resource and bibliography listing titled *Dimensions of Faith and Congregational Ministries with Developmental Disabilities and their Families*. In 1988 the first edition of this book attempted to list all known and available resources in the field of spirituality and disability. It included such topics as theology, worship, religious education, sexuality, congregational awareness, grief, and Jewish resources as well as the names and addresses of faith groups and other agencies providing these and other resources. In 1994 this resource book was produced as a partnership effort between the Division and the Building Community Supports Project at The University Affiliated Program (UAP) of New Jersey, University of Medicine and Dentistry of New Jersey, Robert Wood Johnson Medical School. The coordinator of the project was Bill Gaventa, who at that time was on the staff of The Elizabeth Boggs Center at UMDNJ. In 2001 The Boggs Center took over publication of the book in collaboration with the Division. The full title became *On the Road to Congregational Inclusion: Dimensions of Faith and Congregational Ministries with Persons with Developmental Disabilities and their Families: A Bibliography and Address Listing of Resources for Clergy, Laypersons, Families, and Service Providers*. By 2004 this resource had become a 170-page book which was proving indispensable for persons working in the field of disabilities and spirituality.[8]

EMPOWERING THE PROFESSIONAL

The third major concern of the Religion and Spirituality Division as been the support, nurture, and empowerment of professional religious workers in the field of disabilities, whether they be ordained or lay workers, regardless of faith group. This effort has always sought to reach beyond simply the members of the Division. It has worked to provide resources, networking, and support to those outside the AAMR in order that religion professionals, families of those with disabilities, and others who share the interest in a faith perspective can claim the significance of their work and the importance of sharing spirituality and faith with people with developmental disabilities. Many strategies have already been mentioned in this effort. Two others include the Division's annual Henri Nouwen Award and the Certification Committee.

For many years the AAMR has sought to honor leaders in the fields of research and practice in developmental disabilities. The organization has presented annual awards at its national conference to highlight these individuals and organizations. Following the death of Henri Nouwen in 1996, the Religion and Spirituality Division began talking about an award in his honor which would recognize persons who exemplify Nouwen's concern for persons with disabilities and his leadership in spirituality and practice. In 1997 the Division contacted representatives of the L'Arche community of Daybreak in Toronto, where Henri Nouwen has been pastor for the last ten years of his life. Nathan Bell and Sr. Sue Mosteller gave their approval for such an award. No official AAMR approval was required since the award would be a function of the Division. A committee was appointed to establish the criteria for the award, and the committee called for the first nominations in 2000. The first award was presented in Denver in 2001 during the Division retreat to Sr. Sue Mosteller. Sr. Mosteller had worked with Henri Nouwen during his years at Daybreak and since his death had been serving as executor of his literary estate. Other honorees have included:

- 2002 Virginia "Ginny" Thornburgh, Director, Religion and Disability Program of the NOD
- 2003 James O. Pierson, PhD, Executive Director, Christian Foundation for the Handicapped
- 2004 Charles Luce, Executive Director, National Apostolate for Inclusion Ministry

A second effort in support of religion professionals within the Division focused on certification. Since its inception in the 1960s, the Division leadership had expressed interest in a certification process for chaplains and other religion workers. This interest had led to the organization of the Religious Certification Agency for Retardation (RCAR) in the 1970s. In 1983 Dr. Jack Geistlinger, chair of the RCAR, recommended that the agency be disbanded due to lack of interest and questions about the viability of its processes. In 1984 the Division voted to develop its own certification process, and various people worked on guidelines over a number of years. In 1992 the summer newsletter contained a draft of a certification process for the Division membership to review.

In 1993 at the business meeting during the Washington conference, the Division approved the certification process for persons involved in ordained and pastoral ministries. Dennis Schurter was selected as the first chair of the Certification Committee. Other members were Ingram Parmley, Roger Peters, Elizabeth Sivek, and Fred Stiemke. At the same time, a group was appointed to prepare the certification process for lay religious workers. This committee included Mary Therese Harrington, Julie Hess, Corrine Kavanaugh, and Elizabeth Sivek.

At the 1994 annual meeting Roger Peters was the first member to be certified. In 1995 the Division approved the Code of Ethics for Division members. Certified members were expected to adhere to the Code; for other members the Code was a guideline for voluntary compliance. Fred Stiemke prepared the primary draft of the Code. In 1997 the Division approved the certification process for lay professionals.

The "Continuing Education Guidelines" were approved in 1998. Each certified member was to report at least fifty hours of continuing education activity in order to document one's continuing efforts at professional growth and competency. The certification process and the continuing education guidelines were modeled after those of other organizations such as the Association of Mental Health Clergy and the College of Chaplains (now merged as the Association of Professional Chaplains). At the same time it provided a process that focused on a professional's competencies in ministry with persons with developmental disabilities, resources in that area of ministry, and the flexibility for including lay and ordained, community and institutionally based ministries.

FUTURE DIRECTIONS

The Religion and Spirituality Division's vision for the future primarily focuses on the continued development of its role as a resource organization and support network, advocating for the spiritual lives of people with intellectual and other disabilities. Four areas of emphasis within this vision have found expression in our past and will continue to provide direction for our future.

1. A primary emphasis will be on providing resources and a network for Division members and others within the AAMR to support the spiritual lives of people with disabilities. Networking in new ways will be a challenge as professionals and non-professionals in various fields rely more on the internet and less on national conferences and association meetings for information and professional development. As the costs of association memberships and attendance at national conferences have increased in recent years, it has become more difficult for individuals to belong to multiple organizations and attend conferences in their respective fields. At the same time, non-professionals, lay persons, families, and self-advocates have a growing need for information and support. Even as the Cooperative Resource Exhibit and *On the Road to Congregational Inclusion* continue, the Division will be seeking new avenues for networking and providing resources. Other programs of the Division will also continue to provide support for professional spiritual caregivers, including the Certification Committee and the Henri Nouwen Award.

2. The Division will continue to collaborate and expand its cooperation with other networks and organizations dealing with disability issues, such as groups supporting self-advocates, families, and other religion professionals. Through such collaboration, the Division will seek to strengthen its voice for the spiritual lives of people. Much work needs to be done as ministry with people with disabilities declines in institutional settings and increases in congregational (synagogue, mosque, church) settings. Advocates and self-advocates in local communities need support as they seek to enable congregations to welcome people with disabilities. Collaboration with such groups as the National Organization on Disabilities and The Arc is one way to provide that support.

3. A third emphasis is working with professionals in other fields on the importance of spirituality and spiritual supports as they relate to quality of life, cultural competence, and self-determination. This will take place within the AAMR as the Religion and Spirituality Division relates to other divisions and special interest groups. For example, Division members will be involved with

the Medicine and Gerontology Divisions in addressing issues in healthcare ethics, such as end-of-life concerns. This will also take place through collaborative efforts with other organizations outside of AAMR. One example will be on-going efforts to encourage service providers to assure access to a person's faith tradition and practices for the various people they serve.

4. The Division will continue to work for the integration of disability issues into theological and pastoral education. This will be a continuing effort which has previously found expression in the "Seminary Education" column of the quarterly newsletter. Efforts to integrate one's understanding of the Deity and one's awareness of disabilities is an on-going quest. The Division wants to encourage professionals in the fields of theology and spiritual care to include that quest in their continuing educational programs.

In the forty-five years since Chaplain Don Lawson presented his paper at the AAMD's national convention in Baltimore and gathered three or four other chaplains around him, the Religion and Spirituality Division has journeyed on many paths and climbed many hills in its efforts to nurture the spiritual lives of people with intellectual disabilities, their families, and the professionals who serve them. As the field of intellectual disabilities as changed and the service milieu has broadened, so has changed the vision of the Religion and Spirituality Division in providing resources and support. The members and leaders of the Division look forward to expanding visions of service and support in the years to come.

NOTES

1. The current AAMR divisions include: Administration, Communication Disorders, Community Service, Education, General, Gerontology, Legal Processes & Advocacy, Leisure & Recreation, Medicine, Nursing, Nutrition & Dietetics, OT & PT, Psychology, Religion and Spirituality, Social Work, and Vocational Rehabilitation. Special interest groups (SIG) include: Creative Arts Therapy, Direct Support Professionals, Down Syndrome, Families, Genetics, Health Issues, Mental Health Services, Multicultural Concerns, Sexual/Social Concerns, and Technology. AAMR members are encouraged to express their professional or personal interests by joining one or more of the divisions or SIGs.

2. Information on the early history of the Religion and Spirituality Division comes from Bill Gaventa's article "The Religion Division of the American Association on Mental Retardation" in *The Journal of Pastoral Care*, vol. 42, no. 3, pp. 265-72.

3. At this time the national organization was called the American Association on Mental Deficiency (AAMD). In 1985 it changed its name to the American Association on Mental Retardation (AAMR).

4. Gaventa set forth these proposals as part of a four-page document mailed to the Religion Division membership in the AAMD Religion Division newsletter in January, 1985.

5. This is noted in the 1992 Religion Division Report to the AAMR Board of Directions.

6. A special interest group (SIG) is a group of AAMR members, smaller than a division, focused on special interests such as Down syndrome, families, genetics, sexual/social concerns, and technology.

7. The Division contributed $500; individual members sent donations totaling $1,000.

8. *On the Road to Congregational Inclusion* is currently available for $15 from The Boggs Center, P.O. Box 2688, New Brunswick, NJ 08903. It is also available on the Internet at www.religionaamr.org.

APPENDIX

Religion and Spirituality Division Presidents

1971-73	Ralph Karl
1973-75	
1975-77	Don Lawson
1977-79	Mary Sullivan
1979-81	
1981-83	Ray Chase
1983-85	Bill Gaventa
1985-87	Loren Richter
1987-89	Nancy Lane Chaffee
1989-91	George Decharme
1991-93	Roger Peters
1993-95	Brett Webb-Mitchell
1995-97	Fred Reed
1997-99	Kathryn Jennings
1999-2001	Dennis D. Schurter
2001-03	Vanessa Ervin
2003-05	Garielle Kowolski

The Centennial of Bethesda Lutheran Homes and Services, Inc.

David Morstad, MEd

SUMMARY. Since 1904, Bethesda Lutheran Homes and Services, Inc. has served persons with developmental disabilities. It began as a residential and training under the auspices of Lutheran Church-Missouri Synod and continues today as an expanded national program of residential facilities, group homes, and congregational support for ministries among people with disabilities. While Bethesda has remained faithful to its religious base, it has responded to shifting program emphases in the social arena. In recent years, it has expanded its work to countries of Eastern Europe and elsewhere in order to demonstrate that people with developmental disabilities deserve dignity and respect as God's children. *[Article copies available for a fee from The Haworth Document Delivery Service: 1-800-HAWORTH. E-mail address: <docdelivery@haworthpress.com> Website: <http://www.HaworthPress.com> © 2006 by The Haworth Press, Inc. All rights reserved.]*

KEYWORDS. Bethesda, Lutheran Church-Missouri Synod, residential facilities, group homes, congregational supports

---

David Morstad is Chief Communications Officer for Bethesda Luthern Homes, Inc. In addition to his 28-year career at Bethesda, he is a widely published writer of educational materials for children and adults with developmental disabilities.

[Haworth co-indexing entry note]: "The Centennial of Bethesda Lutheran Homes and Services, Inc." Morstad, David. Co-published simultaneously in *Journal of Religion, Disability & Health* (The Haworth Pastoral Press, an imprint of The Haworth Press, Inc.) Vol. 10, No. 1/2, 2006, pp. 127-140; and: *Disability Advocacy Among Religious Organizations: Histories and Reflections* (ed: Albert A. Herzog, Jr.) The Haworth Pastoral Press, an imprint of The Haworth Press, Inc., 2006, pp. 127-140. Single or multiple copies of this article are available for a fee from The Haworth Document Delivery Service [1-800-HAWORTH, 9:00 a.m. - 5:00 p.m. (EST). E-mail address: docdelivery@ haworthpress.com].

Available online at http://www.haworthpress.com/web/JRDH
© 2006 by The Haworth Press, Inc. All rights reserved.
doi:10.1300/J095v10n01_09

In 2004, three men in Illinois bought a home. They moved into their own house on a quiet street in a medium-sized town–new rooms, new neighbors, new challenges, and responsibilities. While the sense of independence they experienced was that of all new homeowners, there was something distinctive. As men with developmental disabilities, they had for many years received support from Bethesda Lutheran Homes and Services.

Reaching goals that many would find unrealistic or unreachable is more than simply the story of the people Bethesda supports. Since 1904, blessed by God in countless ways, it has been the story of the organization itself.

A recognized service organization of the Lutheran Church-Missouri Synod and a member of Lutheran Services in America, Bethesda Lutheran Homes and Services, Inc. is the oldest Lutheran ministry in the United States serving people with developmental disabilities. From its beginning in Watertown in 1904, Bethesda has grown into one of the most respected organizations in the field.

THE BEGINNING

One hundred years ago, thousands of Americans with developmental disabilities were at the mercy of ignorance and fear. People accepted the popular myths of the time that this disability made people dangerous–even less than completely human. Specialized education, medical treatment and even basic personal care training were rare. There were few schools available that could help individuals with disabilities; few organizations a family could turn to when they were unable to provide the support needed. Religious instruction and support was unusual to find. Lutherans in America took steps to address this situation.[1]

Lutherans who emigrated to the United States identified and organized themselves into synods that reflected their historic ethnicity, U.S. regional settlement and/or particular theological perspectives. The Synodical Conference, organized in Milwaukee in 1872, was a partnership of four synods which were, for the most part, both conservative and predominantly Midwestern. The four groups were: The Lutheran Church-Missouri Synod; the Joint Synod of Wisconsin and Other States; the Slovak Evangelical Lutheran Church of America; and the Norwegian Synod of the American Evangelical Lutheran Church. This Synodical conference formed an organizational base which allowed for the establishment of the Bethesda ministry.

The roots of Bethesda Lutheran Homes and Services can be found in the Lutheran *Kinderfreund* (Children's Friends) societies that were founded throughout the 1800s. These groups were founded primarily to care for orphans although many children who were brought there had disabilities. By the turn of the 20th Century, several of these groups began to organize within the Synodical Conference. They formed the Conference of Lutheran Mission and Charity Associations which included the *Kinderfreund* Societies of Wisconsin, Minnesota, Michigan, Illinois, Iowa, and Missouri and the Lutheran Orphanage Association of Nebraska.[2]

When the Lutheran Church-Missouri Synod held its convention in 1902, leaders from these newly formed charitable organizations proposed that the synod fund a home specifically for people with disabilities. While the church body agreed that the need was great, they felt that it should be funded by private resources rather than the synod. The Synodical Conference later echoed this same sentiment. Undeterred, the *Kinderfreund* Societies made the decision to create the organization on their own.

The initial organizational meeting took place July 7-8, 1903, at Immanuel Lutheran School, Milwaukee. At that time, a letter from William Weiszbrodt, a parochial school teacher near Fall Creek, Wisconsin. was read. He described the progress he had seen at institutions in Europe, particularly the von Bodelschwingh institution in Bethel, Germany. The institution there provided not only homes, daily care and work for those who lived there, but a training center for deacons, deaconesses, nurses and teachers. Most importantly, it had been in operation for more than 50 years at the time and had demonstrated that an endeavor to support people who were "schwachsinnige und epileptishche" ("feeble-minded and epileptic") could be successful.[3] Using The Bethel institution as a pattern, the delegates resolved to form the organization which would, in time, become Bethesda Lutheran Homes and Services. This connection to the facility in Bethel would become rekindled nearly 100 years later in Bethesda's history when an international partnership would lead to assistance efforts in Eastern Europe.[4]

William Weiszbrodt, the school principal who had visited similar facilities in Germany, accepted the call to take charge of the new organization. In keeping with the terminology of the time, it was known as "The Society for the Training and Care of the Feeble Minded and Epileptic." The current name of the organization, "Bethesda" was still nearly 20 years away. Now the questions of the number of people served and location of the organization needed to be addressed.

In order to determine the number of families who might have an interest in the new services, a notice was published in two Lutheran newsletters in the Fall of 1903. The publications, *Der Lutheraner* (Lutheran Church-Missouri Synod) and *Gemindeblatt* (Wisconsin Evangelical Lutheran Synod), encouraged pastors to notify the organization if they knew of needs in their congregations. The number of replies they received was far greater than expected.

In Watertown, Wisconsin, a vacant 45-room structure formerly used as boarding and convalescent space was rented for $55 a month. On April 13, 1904 with five "inmates," as they were referred to at the time, and eight employees, the new organization was begun. Within days, ten more individuals moved in.[5]

The organization continued with its admissions and, two months after its dedication, it was home to 27 people. By December of 1905, all 45 of the rooms at the old Faith Home were occupied.

The board of directors originally set the individual fee for service at $120 a year, but this was soon found to be inadequate. Indeed, other private institutions were known to charge $400-$500. Soon the figure was raised to $200 with parents asked to give more if possible.

Initially, children over 18 years of age were not admitted, nor were those who, in the judgment of the organization, were "proven unfit for training."

The salary of the principal was set at $400 a year, the director at $500 a year, and the janitor, $25 a month.

On July 1, 1905, William Weiszbrodt reported that barely one-fifth of the year's expenses had been covered by payments from the individuals' families. The fact that the treasurer could report a surplus of more than $600 was a tribute to the generous gifts from the organization's supporters.

Then, as now, fundraising was an essential part of the ministry. In early 1905, a few Lutheran pastors became traveling representatives for the organization, calling on individuals and congregations. They collected a building fund of $4,300.

In that same year, though, the owner of the Faith Home building in Watertown refused to renew the organization's lease, setting off a desperate search for new quarters. A three-story frame structure was found on a 2-1/2 acre lot near the northern city limits of Milwaukee. It was the old Riverside Sanitarium and could be leased for 2-1/2 years at $1,300 a year. While it was less suitable than the Watertown location, it would meet the urgent need for space. After a short stay in the parish hall of St. Mark's Lutheran Church in Watertown, the organization packed up and moved to Milwaukee. The move involved people, baggage, records, and all the organization's equipment and supplies, including live cows and chickens.

The Milwaukee location was much smaller than the Faith Home and was terribly crowded. So much so, in fact, 6 girls had to move into the attic of Mr. and Mrs. Weisbrodt's home, across the street. Later, the girls moved back to the main building and 14 boys moved into that same attic. In spite of the crowded conditions, the organization continued its work.

The organization's time in Milwaukee would last less than 3 years, but that era was marked by one very significant event. It was during that time that the organization celebrated its first confirmation. In 1906, at Jerusalem Lutheran Church, five people successfully completed their instruction and together made up the Society's first confirmation class.

From a traditional Lutheran perspective, the rite of Confirmation is a significant aspect of Christian life. Indeed, for much of the early history of the organization one of the principal purposes of admission was to reach this goal. Confirmation is at its core a reaffirmation of the vows made by parents and godparents (sponsors) at the time of infant baptism. In the non-disabled population it has traditionally occurred among middle school aged children following a two- to three-year period of study highlighting Martin Luther's writings on the Ten Commandments, the Lord's Prayer, the Creeds and related scripture. Perhaps because of its very academic tradition, Confirmation of individuals with disabilities was a landmark event in the early 20th Century and remains an area of great interest among Lutheran clergy to this day.

HOME TO WATERTOWN

In 1909, faced with the crowded conditions in Milwaukee and a growing waiting list for services, the Board of Directors decided to build larger quarters–enough to serve 85 people. It was decided that the best option was to erect this new building back where things began, in Watertown, where they still owned land donated in 1903 by Heinrich Klug.

The land that Klug donated was located on the banks of the Rock River on the northern edge of the city. However, the ignorance of disabilities that prevailed at the time was about to show itself in a profound way. Some of the citizens of Watertown objected to the organization's use of that parcel of land. Their belief was that this type of disability was contagious. They feared that since the river ran through this particular piece of land and then flowed through the rest of the city, there was a chance that the water itself could be somehow contaminated, posing a danger to the rest of the city's population.

These irrational worries convinced the organization to trade that land for a different parcel, also located on the Rock River, but on the southwest side of the city. On a warm Sunday afternoon in June of 1909, members of the Society and hundreds of visitors gathered in Watertown as the cornerstone for the new building was laid.[6]

The new home was a very simple structure–the first and second floors were bedrooms and living rooms, and the sunny spaces on the third floor became schoolrooms. Partly because the construction provided even more visibility and awareness of the organization, admissions continued at a startling rate. The new quarters at Watertown were filled almost as soon as they became available.

Less than one year after the dedication of the new building in Watertown, acting Superintendent Louis Pingel reported an enrollment of 75 individuals. Pingel had become the first director in February of 1908 and remained until August of 1915. He returned to Bethesda in 1921 and stayed until his retirement in 1945. In spite of the official designation of "superintendent," Pingel's responsibilities were, of necessity, broad. They included teaching, recreation, equipment maintenance, and occasional care of the livestock.

In keeping with the character of rural Wisconsin at that time, the original Bethesda homestead was in fact a working farm that provided jobs, produce and income for the organization. It was a central part of everyday life at Bethesda for the first 50 years of its existence. Vegetables were preserved; milk was sold; and the men, women, boys, and girls who were supported there found purpose and value in their labor that they may not have found elsewhere. The farm operation also helped develop friendships with the people and the merchants in the area. One example of this was recorded on Christmas of 1911. Louis Pingel had gone from person to person preparing a list of all their Christmas wishes and the list was then taken to area stores. Merchants commonly provided the goods at no charge. One provided a cash donation besides.

In 1913, the enrollment passed the 100 mark and continued to rise. The farm was too small to adequately provide for all. The kitchen, dining room, and schoolrooms were all overcrowded. The Board of Directors once again looked to expand.

One particular passage from the Gospel of John became an inspiration for the organization: "After this there was a feast of the Jews, and Jesus went up to Jerusalem. Now there is in Jerusalem by the Sheep Gate a pool, in Hebrew called Bethesda, which has five porticoes. In these lay a multitude of invalids, blind, lame, paralyzed. One man was there, who had been ill for thirty-eight years. When Jesus saw him and knew that he had been lying there a long time, he said to him, "Do you want to be healed?" The sick man answered him, "Sir, I have no man to put me into the pool when the water is troubled, and while I am going another steps down before me." Jesus said to him, 'Rise, take up your pallet, and walk.' And at once the man was healed, and he took up his pallet and walked" (John 5:1-8).[7]

This story was so meaningful that when the new building erected upon the return to Watertown, one word—"Bethesda," which means "House of Mercy"—was placed above the main entrance. And finally, in 1923, the name of the organization was officially changed to *Bethesda Lutheran Home.*[8]

At the time of the organization's move to Watertown, the society was still in its infancy and struggling to keep its head above water. Besides the ever-present shortage of funds, there were other difficulties. Bethesda was almost always understaffed. The monthly salary at the time was $35 plus room and board. For several periods in 1920, a staff of 4 employees was responsible for almost 150 people—day and night.

More and more people were learning about the church's work at Bethesda, however, and thus the organization and the individuals themselves were constantly making new friends. Something that helped greatly was the publication of a small quarterly paper titled "Der Bote Aus Bethesda" (The Bethesda Messenger). Since the early supporters of Bethesda were mainly Lutherans of German ancestry, at least part of the Messenger was printed in German until 1942. At first, the newsletter was dedicated mainly to appeals and pleas for necessary items such as food and clothing, as well as wheelchairs, pianos, shoes, sheets, towels and wash cloths that were needed by the organization. The publication gradually became a useful informational tool in providing information about the organization to church congregations in the area as Bethesda tried to increase its number of supporters.

In the 1920s, the Associated Lutheran Charities recommended that the Deaconess Association open a training school for nurses at Bethesda. The Bethesda Messenger encouraged women between 18 and 35 to "come serve the Lord with gladness." The Deaconess Association promised to furnish uniforms, a modest allowance of spending money, and care in sickness and old age. In all, 14 young women came to Bethesda for 2 years to work and be trained as nurses. They received training and graduated in May of 1927.[9]

From the move back to Watertown in 1909, through the next 30 years, the shape of the organization continually changed. Buildings were erected to accommodate the ever growing population. More people meant a greater need for farmland and so 80 more acres were added in 1919. By 1929, Bethesda was home to 320 individuals.

THE WAR YEARS

While the Great Depression affected everyone—including those people living in rural Watertown, WI, the focus of Bethesda's mission and ministry remained strong. In May of 1935, a very special cornerstone was laid. One year later, the new Chapel at Bethesda was formally dedicated. It was the perfect place for morning and evening devotions and Sunday worship services, and quickly became the centerpiece of the organization. It seemed a fitting symbol for the organization, since the teaching of God's Word was, and still is, the centerpiece of the services and supports offered by Bethesda.

Soon after the Great Depression had ended, the United States found itself in the middle of another World War. The war years meant shortages of food, fuel, and workers. During this time Bethesda was running on borrowed money. Wages at Bethesda were relatively low in comparison to factories. Twelve-hour shifts were the norm at the time, and most of the staff worked seven days a week. Some had no days off for a two or three-year time period.

It is often in times of adversity that people step forward in selfless ways and such was the case at this time of Bethesda's history. Sensing the future of the organization and those people it supported was at stake, the loyal employees of the organization requested a 10-percent pay cut. Later the Board was forced to reduce wages even more. Unfortunately, the deaconess school languished during this period and finally closed its doors.

As the depression continued, new sources of revenue were found. When the sheep were sheared, the wool batts were sold for quilts at $3 per batt. Thistle tea, "good for rheumatism and other ailments," according to the Bethesda Messenger, also was sold. The wild Canada thistle was picked from roadsides, washed in rainwater, dried on racks and then ground and sold for $1 per pound.

The 1940s were a period of careful spending, to be sure, but by 1950, almost $400,000 worth of remodeling had been completed. It included a new office wing, a second elevator, a fireproof stairway with iron steps, and numerous improvements for the farm operation. Interest from families continued to be strong and Bethesda was again poised for expansion.

A new building–enough to accommodate 150 people–was contemplated but as it was reported by the superintendent at the time, "A new building will bring 150 more persons to be fed three times daily. That will demand either increasing our present farm acreage or spending an increasing amount of money to buy groceries and produce. Naturally, a completed new building will not run itself but will have to be staffed. But where and how to get all these workers when we don't have nearly enough for our present plant and can't seem to engage any!"[10]

In 1950, as the organization contemplated the challenges ahead, Rev. Clarence Golisch took the position of superintendent. He did not hesitate to build and remodel to accommodate more individuals. Under his guidance, the population served by the organization increased from 320 to 660. Also, staff hours were decreased to 8-hour days and wages were increased.

Dr. Golisch was a leader of both vision and commitment. As early as 1952 he reported, "The trend in secular circles is away from institutions, even though many states are building larger and improved such facilities. I believe the trend is in the right direction to provide community facilities for retaining these children in normal channels of living as much as possible." Consequently, Bethesda's first community-based group home was established in Watertown in 1961. Clarence Golisch served Bethesda until his retirement in 1972.

CHALLENGES OF THE MODERN AGE

The era of the 1960s and 70s were a time of great cultural change in the United States. The attention drawn to civil rights concerns had an unintended benefit to people with disabilities. People were beginning to recognize the need for growth, learning, and freedom for all people–including those with disabilities.[11]

While Bethesda had faced difficult times in the past, they had always been due to funding, space and related internal concerns. A set of challenges that occurred in the early 70s were something new. Regulatory agencies were now being called upon to look with much greater scrutiny at facilities such as Bethesda. As a result, the organization which had operated as a reasonably successful self-sufficient community of happy individuals for nearly 70 years now found itself with 238 separate deficiencies in state codes–most having to do with record-keeping, living area design, and education for the residents. The seemingly strong and healthy organization was now at the point of near closure and the need for a new type of leadership could not have been clearer.

In order to deal with these immediate challenges and set the organization on a new course for the future, the board of directors hired Alexander L. Napolitano as its new executive director in 1975. A business administration graduate of Fairleigh Dickinson University, Napolitano also had a master's degree in health care administration from George Washington University, and additional coursework at Rutgers University. His experience included hospital and mental health care administration and he was skilled in dealing with legislative requirements.

The immediate improvements initiated by Napolitano helped save Bethesda from serious penalties and perhaps closure, but it was his continued strong leadership that led the organization into a new era of expansion, outreach and fiscal strength. Before his retirement in 1997, Napolitano received and honorary doctorate from Concordia University and was appointed to the President's Committee on Mental Retardation.

Under Napolitano's leadership, a new emphasis was placed on education and training programs, vocational opportunities, and greater community involvement. There was a substantial addition of teaching and nursing staff at Bethesda, and the addition of a full-time medical director.

While Bethesda had served families from throughout the United States, it had always done so from its facilities in Wisconsin. In the 70s, the time had come to step beyond Watertown to other parts of the country. Bethesda's first out-of-state group home opened in Maryville, Missouri, in 1977. From there, the Bethesda family would expand over the next 20 years to Illinois, Indiana, Florida, Michigan, Ohio, Texas, Kansas, New Jersey, and beyond.

THE BIRTH OF OUTREACH SERVICES

By 1980, the face of developmental disabilities in the United States was changing. Medical advancements were improving, and sometimes saving lives; laws were in place to guarantee public education to all children, regardless of any disability; parents were both informed and strong advocates for their loved ones. The result was that more and more people wanted advice about their personal situations, referrals to services in their own home towns and resources they could use in their own homes, churches and communities. With 80 years of experience to offer, Bethesda stepped forward to establish the National Christian Resource Center in 1985. The NCRC, as it is commonly called, provides information to parents, and curriculum materials and teacher training for congregations.

The NCRC also produces staff training materials for professionals who work for other agencies in the field. Each year, thousands of people benefit from Bethesda's experience, leadership, and Christian values.

As a result of the expanding organization and the new roles that Bethesda Lutheran Home was playing in terms of outreach to others, the name of the organization was changed in 1992 to Bethesda Lutheran Homes and Services, Inc.

BETHESDA TODAY

Today, people with disabilities need places to live, work, worship and play. Bethesda Lutheran Homes and Services seeks to provide comfortable homes, supportive partners, training, and advocacy within an atmosphere of Christian love and caring. At this writing, late in 2004, Bethesda is providing direct support to 1,100 individuals in a wide variety of residential settings in thirteen states.

Pastors, teachers, and parents turn to Bethesda for assistance in developing special needs ministry programs in their own congregations. In an effort to directly assist them, Bethesda created several Parish Ministry Consultant (PMC) positions throughout the US. PMC's provide advocacy, information, teaching tools, training, and encouragement to all those involved in special needs ministry at the congregational level.

Today, citizens with developmental disabilities are partners in planning their own lives, full of their own hopes, dreams, and accomplishments.

INTERNATIONAL EFFORTS

In 2003, Bethesda joined with other Lutheran agencies to create IMPACT, an alliance that provides assistance to non-governmental organizations who work with people with disabilities in Latvia, Eastern Europe, and other countries around the world. The other member agencies include Mosaic, Bethphage Great Britain, the Deacony Foundation of Northern Norway and the von Bodelschwingh institution of Bethel, Germany–the same organization that inspired the formation of Bethesda at the beginning of the 20th century. IMPACT afforded Bethesda the opportunity to make its first effort to directly support individuals outside the United States in Romania.

The deplorable conditions of the orphanages in Romania have been well documented in the national media. An ABC news broadcast in the late 1990s displayed graphic images of neglect and mistreatment. The rate of child abandonment is high and conditions for children with developmental disabilities appear as hopeless as anyone could imagine. As part of the IMPACT partnership, representatives from Bethesda traveled to Bucharest in 2002 to provide staff training and make plans to move children with developmental disabilities to safer and more loving environments. In the spring of 2003, Bethesda helped move the first four children to their new home. Since then, three group homes have been constructed, providing a new life for 22 children with developmental disabilities.

E-mail received from a Bethesda staff person on her first visit to Romania included the following observations:

> *The orphanage is probably as you imagine. The noise and smell can be overwhelming at times and there is no air. There are several large rooms with rows of beds and one large dining room. . . . We found many children with scars covering their body. Several had open wounds. One little boy I spent time with had bruises covering most of his back. All are starved for love and attention. We try to spend time at each visit just playing, holding and hugging children. . . . Today I saw a very young boy, about 8-9-years-old lying in a doorway of a building. He was curled up in a ball in the corner. His arms were pulled into his shirt for warmth and the edge of his collar pulled up over his ears. His little head was lying on the hard, rough concrete. . . . There are hundreds of children living in the sewers of Bucharest.*

Other international programs currently in operation include Latvia, Nizhney Novgorod, in western Russia, and the Home of New Hope in the Dominican Republic.

At the dawn of its second century, even the Watertown, Wisconsin campus has taken on a newly remodeled look. Spaces that are comfortable, personal and attractive announce to all who visit that the founding principles of Bethesda are still honored–that people with disabilities, created and redeemed by God, are worthy of dignity and respect.

From its humble beginnings through periods of growth and struggle, one thing has remained constant at Bethesda–the organization's mission to provide quality Christ-centered services and supports to people with developmental disabilities. And it is that mission, along with the experience of past successes that Bethesda will take into its second century of service.

FUTURE CHALLENGES

Two challenges in particular appear on the horizon for the organization–challenges faced by all support providers in the field. One issue that has remained constant throughout Bethesda's history is the concern over how the mission will be funded. In the early years, the funding source was a combination of charitable resources and agricultural self-support. Today, a different combination exists. Government funding in a variety of sources provides the majority of support but is insufficient to meet the level of quality to which the organization remains committed. Individual contributions continue to feed an investment effort that makes up the difference between government funding and the ongoing cost of operation. The funding challenges in the future are clear. Government funding for developmental disability services has been reduced in nearly every state and there is a critical need for strong advocacy among policy makers.[12]

A second issue that emerges is that of Bethesda's response to the self-advocate. Historically, the strongest voices for people with disabilities have been families and other advocates. Like all responsible providers, Bethesda must continue to seek ways to hear and respond to the voices and choices of the individuals who have developmental disabilities. Only when the hopes and dreams of those with the most intense disabilities are as fully realized as those of non-disabled people will the vision of Bethesda's founders be fulfilled.

Some profound truths have been discovered in the past 100 years, and this much is known: As we reach out and offer support to people with disabilities, we discover the rich blessings they have to share in return.

NOTES

1. Taege, M. (1979). *Why are they so happy?* Bethesda Lutheran Homes and Services. 29-30.
2. Taege, M. (1979). 27-28.

3. Bradfield, M. (1964). *City of Mercy: The Story of Bethel*. Verlagshandlung der Anstalt Bethel. 15-16.

4. About IMPACT. (2004). Global advocacy for people with disabilities. http://www. impact-the-world.org

5. Taege, M. (1979). 30.

6. Watertown Historical Society. (2002). *A History of Watertown, WI*.

7. Revised Standard Version. University of Virginia.

8. Der Bote aus Bethesda. (1923). Bethesda Lutheran Homes and Services.

9. Fritschel, H. (1949). *A Story of One Hundred Years of Deaconess Service: By the Institution of Protestant Deaconesses, Pennsylvania, and the Lutheran Deaconess Motherhouse at Milwaukee, Wisconsin 1849-1949. Milwaukee: Lutheran Deaconess Motherhouse.*

10. Report of the superintendent to the Bethesda Board of Directors. 1949.

11. Patton, J., & Payne, J. (1990). *Mental Retardation*. Columbus, OH. Merrill Publishing Company. 21-22.

12. Braddock, D. (Ed.). (2002). *Disability at the dawn of the 21st century and the state of the states*. Washington, DC: American Association on Mental Retardation.

The Christian Council
on Persons with Disabilities:
Goals Network, Encourage, Impact

Marlys Taege, PhB, LittD

SUMMARY. The Christian Council on Persons with Disabilities (CCPD) is a unique organization because it encompasses all disabilities–physical, mental, developmental, hearing, visual, learning, and environmental. Founded by Joni Eareckson Tada to provide a united voice for Christian disability ministries in North America, it has achieved significant accomplishments in advocacy, networking, and training through its conferences, awards, publications, speakers, mentoring, and services. Its newest emphasis is CCPD CAN (Connecting, Advancing and Nurturing disability ministries). *[Article copies available for a fee from The Haworth Document Delivery Service: 1-800-HAWORTH. E-mail address: <docdelivery@ haworthpress.com> Website: <http://www.HaworthPress.com> © 2006 by The Haworth Press, Inc. All rights reserved.]*

KEYWORDS. Disabilities, disability ministry, CCPD, accessibility, inclusion, Christian Council, advocacy, disability awards

Marlys Taege, who worked for Bethesda Lutheran Home and Services and served as Executive Director of the Christian Council on Persons with Disabilities, is currently a writer living in Wisconsin.

[Haworth co-indexing entry note]: "The Christian Council on Persons with Disabilities Goals: Network, Encourage, Impact" Taege, Marlys. Co-published simultaneously in *Journal of Religion, Disability & Health* (The Haworth Pastoral Press, an imprint of The Haworth Press, Inc.) Vol. 10, No. 1/2, 2006, pp. 141-162; and: *Disability Advocacy Among Religious Organizations: Histories and Reflections* (ed: Albert A. Herzog, Jr.) The Haworth Pastoral Press, an imprint of The Haworth Press, Inc., 2006, pp. 141-162. Single or multiple copies of this article are available for a fee from The Haworth Document Delivery Service [1-800-HAWORTH, 9:00 a.m. - 5:00 p.m. (EST). E-mail address: docdelivery@haworthpress.com].

As people with disabilities have struggled to achieve the basics of life enjoyed by temporarily able-bodied citizens, they have also developed a determination to use their experience for the benefit of others. As a result, numerous Christian ministries, headed by individuals who had overcome obstacles to inclusion in education, employment, recreation and Christian churches, had sprung up across the United States by the 1980s.

Scattered and struggling to expand their programs, these disability ministry organizations were dedicated to advocacy, inclusion, and service. Although supported by families and friends, their leaders were working in isolation with little knowledge of what similar groups across the country were achieving and without the impact of a unified Christian voice at the national level.

To bring these individuals together, Joni and Friends, the disability ministry of Joni Eareckson Tada, sponsored the National Congress on the Church and the Disabled in 1988 on the campus of Wheaton College in Wheaton, Illinois. Over 700 people with disabilities, advocates, family members, friends, and disability ministry workers participated. They came from across the country to gain fresh information, develop new skills, and create a network that would not only benefit members but also enable its leaders to impact governmental entities and the Christian church at large.

During this historic event, 30 key leaders in the Christian disability community met at Tada's invitation to develop an action plan. She thought a strong voice was needed to get the attention of national leaders and encourage them to work in the area of disabilities. That, she believed, could come only from a united front. Her guests agreed that uniting under a shared vision and common goals would further advance Christ's gospel in the disability community–and thus was born the Christian Council on Persons with Disabilities (CCPD).

Twelve board members were selected (later increased to 18), and Tada became its first president. An office was established at the headquarters of one of CCPD's founding members, the Christian League for the Handicapped (today known as Inspiration Ministries), Walworth, Wisconsin. Its executive director, Steve Jensen, served as CCPD's first vice-president and later as its second president.

Chartered in the State of Wisconsin, the new organization received tax-exempt status in March 1989 and began work immediately. Tada and Jensen laid plans to gain the attention of church leadership through publicity, position papers, magazine articles, and press interviews.

The purpose of the new organization according to the Bylaws was to (1) promote the biblical perspective on persons with disabilities and the church; (2) offer the church an evangelical position on issues related to disabilities; (3) establish standards that will advance the ministry gifts of persons with disabilities; and (4) encourage Christian leaders to take initiatives that will enable persons with disabilities to actively and fully participate in the life and ministry of the church.

Unlike most Christian disability ministries that focus on the particular disability or interest of the founder(s), CCPD was unique because it encompassed all disabilities–physical, mental, developmental, visual, hearing, learning, and environmental.

PRINCIPLES OF MINISTRY ADOPTED

The Board adopted the Statement of Faith of the National Association of Evangelicals (NAE) and determined that membership in CCPD would be "open to individuals and organizations that support our evangelical Statement of Faith." To apply that statement more specifically to disability ministry, the Board later adopted these "Principles of Ministry" written by a board member, Dr. Thomas B. Hoeksema of Calvin College:

> *CCPD believes that God is Creator, Redeemer, and the Lord of all creation.* Specifically we confess:

1. That all people are made in God's image in order to serve Him in all the arenas of life.
2. That human life has become broken through sin, and one of sin's consequences is suffering.
3. That Christ bears our griefs, carries our sorrows, and heals our brokenness in body and spirit.
4. That in order to live fully, now and forever, we must have a personal faith in Jesus as Savior.
5. That we are called to personal salvation *and* a life of thankful and obedient response.

> *Our confession has at least the following implications:*

1. Christ clearly teaches the sanctity of life, no matter how severe the disabling condition.

2. Christ's example and the law of love demand that we compassionately respond to the needs of persons who have disabilities and to
   their families; we must walk together in our suffering.
3. We must remove any architectural, attitudinal or communication
   barriers that impede the message of salvation or hinder the participation of any person in the life of the church.
4. We must enable the spiritual, intellectual, social, emotional, and
   physical development of all persons so they may be faithful stew-
   ards of the gifts God has given and may respond obediently to
   God's call of discipleship.
5. We must make public the gifts of people whom society defines as
   disabled, so they may participate mutually in our interdependent
   family.

ADVOCACY AND EDUCATION EFFORTS INITIATED

To launch its advocacy on the national level, CCPD leaders introduced a resolution on the church and disability at the 1989 annual convention of the National Association of Evangelicals. A presentation to
the NAE board by CCPD leaders won support and led to subsequent
passage at the NAE membership meeting. The resolution encouraged
churches to welcome and include persons with disabilities in their planning and programs.

In May 1989, CCPD sponsored a "Symposium on Disability and the
Church" at Inspiration Center, Walworth, Wisconsin. Disability Ministry
representatives met to develop position papers on key disability concerns
relative to the church. These included *Church Attitude and Responsibility*, *The Role and Responsibility of the Pastor*, *Everyday Accessibility*,
Political Issues, and *Evangelism, Discipleship and Missions*.

For the rest of the year, CCPD efforts focused on informing the
Christian community about the Americans with Disabilities Act. Articles by CCPD leaders appeared in such magazines as *Christianity Today*, *Contact* (for the Christian Businessmen's Committee), *Journal of
Christian Camping*, and *Positive Approach*. Tada, Jensen, and other
board members were interviewed on their local radio stations as well as
national networks, including "Focus on the Family News" and "Family
Radio."

In May 1990, CCPD joined Joni and Friends in co-sponsoring the "International Congress on Church and Disability." Over 600 disability

workers from 38 states and 39 foreign countries attended this educational and inspirational event at Calvin College in Grand Rapids, Michigan.

NO CONSENSUS ATTAINED

From then until 2004, CCPD sponsored annual educational conferences.

A symposium format was used in 1991 at Inspiration Center, with Steve Estes, author of *Called to Die* and *A Step Further*, as guest speaker. The program addressed the issue of job access in Christian businesses and churches, but participants also raised questions regarding life issues,

Euthanasia therefore was chosen as the subject of the 1992 symposium at Sandy Cove Bible Conference Center in northeast Maryland. Presenters included Dr. Bud Bouma of Calvin College's biology department, Dr. David Biebel, editor of *Physician Magazine*, published by "Focus on the Family," and Joni Eareckson Tada.

Strong discussions followed the presentations at both conferences, but the unified voice sought by CCPD leaders on issues relating to employment laws and initiatives, quality of life, and euthanasia concerns was not achieved. It quickly became apparent that Christians with disabilities, like everyone else, enjoy the option of adopting different perspectives regarding proposed laws and governmental involvement in everyday life.

Because CCPD leaders then realized they could not speak with a single voice for all members and member organizations, their primary concentration became training and networking for disability ministry leaders and advocates. Nevertheless, the Council continued to impact public opinion and the lives of people who have disabilities through its conferences, awards, newsletter, Christian service and outreach.

CONFERENCES TACKLE CHALLENGING ISSUES

Subsequently, as each annual conference explored a different disability ministry concern, attendance increased, and participants enjoyed the expanding opportunities for networking.

A symposium on "Life Worth Living" was held in 1993 at Arrowhead Springs Conference Center, San Bernardino, California. Joni Eareckson

Tada spoke on "Quality of Life." Breakout sessions covered such subjects as Circles of Support, Mainstreaming, Camping, Supported Living Arrangements, and the Biblical Basis for Disability Ministry.

CCPD's annual gathering in 1994 was held in conjunction with JAF Ministries' "Institute on The Church and Disability" in Knoxville, Tennessee. The week-long event was designed to provide intense training for leaders and potential leaders on the Christian response to needs and opportunities within the disability community. The Institute coincided with a "Meet the Challenge" Ability Expo sponsored by the Christian Federation for the Handicapped.

The week included an evening at Johnson Bible College, where Tada spoke on "Establishing a Theological Framework for Ministry." The college was in the process of establishing a minor in disability ministry under the leadership of Jim Pierson, a CCPD board member.

"Independence versus Rebellion" was the focus of CCPD's 1995 conference at Park Avenue Baptist Church, Titusville, Florida. Pre-conference publicity noted, "As more and more people who are mentally challenged are reaching out for independence, some of our church members are stepping over the line into rebellion against parents, against traditions, and against the church. There is a growing need to help those in the mentally challenged community who are being empowered with independence as well as to exhort them against the allure of rebellion. We will wrestle together with this timely issue."

Conference planners saw rebellion in many forms: Paul and Marie wanted to get married; their parents did not agree, yet professionals said the couple should exercise their right. Andy wanted to have his own apartment; his mother was opposed and had legitimate safety concerns. John, a group home resident, also wanted his own apartment. His new residence would be across town in an unsafe area. His father was concerned because he had fought hard for John's group home placement, and there might not be one in the future if/when needed. In all three cases, the people looked to their church for help, and the pastors were struggling to find the right answers.

Integration and mainstreaming were the focus of the 1996 conference in Grand Rapids, Michigan, under the theme, "That All May Serve." "More Than an Address," the 1997 conference at Mt. Gilead Camp in California stressed housing options for people with disabilities and provided sessions on board development and ministry trends. "Evangelizing and Discipling Persons Who Have Disabilities" was the emphasis in 1997 at Titusville, Florida.

To encourage their involvement in disability ministry, a luncheon for pastors preceded the 10th anniversary conference in Indianapolis, Indiana, in 1998. At the opening session, Ginny Thornburgh of the National Organization on Disability (NOD) announced its Accessible Congregations Campaign, whose goal was to gain the commitment of 2,000 congregations by the year 2000 to include people with all types of disabilities as full and active participants. CCPD became a co-sponsor of the campaign.

At the "Ministering Hand in Hand" conference in 1999 in Milwaukee, Wisconsin, the Rev. D. Cordell Brown spoke from his experience as a person with cerebral palsy when he challenged participants, "If you are really going to be leaders in the disability community, then you've really got to love them . . . love them lavishly . . . love them with all your heart. . . . I don't care how many curb cuts you have or how many ramps you make to your platform. I don't care how accessible your bathrooms are . . . how many pew cuts you have–whether in front or back or halfway in-between. But what I do care about is that each disabled person is a real part of your congregation . . . is really loved!"

Dr. Robertson McQuilkin gave the keynote address at the 2000 conference in Colorado Springs, Colorado. He had retired after 22 years as president of Columbia (South Carolina) International University to care for his wife Muriel when she developed Alzheimer's Disease. His theme was "2000 and Beyond–Disability Ministry in a New Millennium." He asked,

> What if we changed 'disabled' to 'limited ability'? That's all of us! . . . We live in a fallen world, and the Christian is not exempt. If that were not so, everyone would be a Christian–but what kind? We need to get real–God does not promise to shield or intervene. The prosperity gospel is not good news–it leads to the sin of unbelief. We don't get an automatic pass in this fallen world!

Other speakers offered help on "Remaining Christian while Working within the System" and "Coloring Outside the Lines" (i.e.,"Christians Must Embrace Innovation").

In 2001, CCPD met in Fullerton, California, to hear Doug Mazza, executive vice president of JAF Ministries, discuss "Gaining Power by Surrendering Control." A former automotive executive, he is the father of a severely disabled son. Joni Eareckson Tada also spoke on "Strength for the Journey." Opening with a concert by Renee Bondi, a quadriplegic Gospel singer, the gathering drew 284 attendees, evidence of the growing popularity of CCPD's annual conferences.

Describing her discussion with an AIDS victim who did not know the Lord, Joni commented, "Some would say I should have grabbed him by the shirt collar, shoved the 'Four Spiritual Laws' down his throat, and left tracts on his bedside." But, she explained,

> Long ago I realized that there is no nuclear weapon of evangelism that explodes people out of the water and gets them into the Gospel boat. There is no atomic bomb that is going to flatten people's resistance. NO! A person usually comes to Christ having picked up bits and pieces of the Gospel here and there along the way. Nudged forward, they move sideways. They go laterally until finally under the pressure of the power of everybody else's prayers, their heart warms and they are open to the truth.

Joni challenged her audience, "Will you realign your ministry's priorities and the priority of disability outreach in your church, so that it is not only to demonstrate the love of Christ through meeting practical needs, but to declare the love of Christ to the perishing?"

Under the bold theme, "Expanding the Horizons–The Sky Is Not the Limit!" the 2002 conference in Orlando, Florida, opened with a concert by Gospel singer and song-writer Tony Elenburg of Nashville. Demonstrating his positive approach to his trials with polio, Tony said, "It's all a matter of perspective–I'm not limping; everyone else is!"

Keynote speaker Dr. H. Norman Wright, therapist, pastor and author of over 60 books, spoke from his experience as the father of a disabled son. "Don't try to go it alone," he urged, but "make sure people around you are supportive." He identified the five major loss events of life as death, divorce, diagnosis (of a serious illness), disability and disappointment (example: job loss). With disability, he noted, there is no ritual to commemorate the loss, grief is chronic, and there is no distinguishing between the person and the condition. "You become the condition. . . . We must educate people!"

Because no Christian camping association was giving priority to inclusion and accessibility, CCPD President Don Crooker convened a pre-conference gathering in 2002 for directors and staffs of Christian camps that serve people with disabilities. Reaction was so positive that it became a yearly event covering everything from forms and funding to programming and communicating spiritual truths.

Sue Thomas, the inspiration for the TV show, "Sue Thomas: F.B.Eye," opened the 2003 conference in Lisle, Illinois. Profoundly deaf from the age of 18 months, she shared how she had "worked all my life to function in the hearing world." Her hard work paid off when she was hired by the Federal Bureau of Investigation in Washington, DC. Because of her superb ability to read lips, she was soon doing undercover surveillance. After her FBI career, she studied at the Columbia International University Graduate School in Bible and Missions and became a popular Christian speaker.

Under the theme, "That All May Live," this 15th anniversary conference focused on medical-ethical issues with Dr. Nigel Cameron as the main speaker. The executive chairman of the Center for Bioethics and Public Policy in London, England, and the Center for Bioethics and Culture, Oakland, California, he had gained considerable renown through his "debate of the century" with Peter Singer on the subject, "What Does It Mean to Be Human?" A Princeton University professor, Singer was known for his support of euthanasia for disabled children and infirm adults.

A third speaker, Chris Ralston, whose disability was the result of his mother having Rubella while pregnant with him, discussed "Disability and Suffering" and "End of Life Care." At the time he was studying for a master's degree in bioethics at Trinity International University, Deerfield, Illinois.

Keynote speaker for the 2004 educational conference in Indianapolis was Bill Gaventa, Director of Community and Congregational Supports at the Elizabeth M. Boggs Center on Developmental Disabilities in New Jersey and Executive Secretary of the Religion and Spirituality Division of the American Association on Mental Retardation. The theme was "That All May Serve." Pianist and singer Ginny Owens, blind since age two and a Dove Award winner, gave the opening concert.

Supporting person-centered planning, Gaventa urged his audience to "Help everybody discover their gifts. . . . Assess their strengths and interests." He noted that the root of the word "assess" implies "sit next to." So, he concluded, "Don't just do something–be there!"

IMPACTING LIVES THROUGH SERVICES

With the Americans with Disabilities Act bringing disability issues to the forefront during CCPD's early years, and with right-to-die legislation proposed in California, Iowa, Oklahoma, Michigan, Colorado,

Florida, and New Hampshire, the Council received numerous *media opportunities*. During the first half of 1992, CCPD leaders were involved in nearly 50 interviews on Christian radio across the country, including one on CBN.

As added services, a *mentoring program* was launched and *an electronic bulletin board* established in 1994. Board member Steve Kranz monitored the bulletin board from the office of his ministry, Oaks of Hebron in Rohnert Park, California.

Meanwhile, the CCPD office was linked to the Internet, allowing Marlys Taege, the new executive director, to answer disability questions posted on various discussion pages and to connect via e-mail with people from around the world who were seeking resources for disability ministry. A CCPD Website was established in 1997 and redesigned in 2000.

Starting in 2000, efforts were made to develop a *Speakers' Bureau*, and work was begun on a position paper about "The Value of Life." Two previous position papers covered "A Person's Worth and Work" and "Euthanasia."

Through *displays and presentations* at Christian conferences and disability awareness events, CCPD educated thousands of young people and adults on the importance of including people with disabilities in Christian churches and friendships. Among the conferences at which CCPD members staffed displays were Urbana 2000 (Intervarsity Christian Fellowship); the Moody Missions conference (CCPD's executive director and two members led workshops and interacted with students heading for the mission field); McLean Bible Church's Access Summit in McLean, Virginia; various NOD "That All May Worship" conferences; and events sponsored by the National Council of Christian Churches Committee on Disabilities. CCPD's executive director annually reported on its accomplishments and plans at the committee meetings.

Because church members tend to be frightened by the lengthy *accessibility surveys* published by some disability organizations, CCPD developed a simpler review that included an easy-to-understand rationale for its questions. The introduction explained that "with 19% of the U.S. population having some type of disability and considering all the family members who impacted by a relative's disability, it becomes obvious that church accessibility (both attitudinal and architectural) is an important factor in reaching people who do not know Christ."

It also noted that "most of us may eventually have difficulty walking, seeing or hearing, so accommodations (such as ramps) can also be a blessing for many in the church, including parents of small children." In addition, it pointed out that meeting most of the needs of people with disabilities did not have to be expensive. Entitled "How Accessible Is Our Church?" the survey was well received and used extensively. It is available on the CCPD Website (www.ccpd.org).

CCPD's *first regional chapter* was established in South Wisconsin in 1995. It held several successful meetings but dissolved a couple years later when leaders lacked the time to continue. (Most CCPD members have always been heavily involved in the disability ministry of their own organization, their church, or their employer, so they have little time to serve in additional capacities. Their primary fund-raising allegiance also has been to their own organization.) A second regional chapter organized in California in 1996 also was discontinued after a short time because several other disability organizations were holding conferences and regular meetings there. Periodically CCPD received other requests for chapters, but its guidelines required that there always be a board member mentor for a new chapter, so when none was available, new chapters could not materialize.

At the request of the Home of Eternal Love (an orphanage serving discarded handicapped children) in Xi'an, China, CCPD *coordinated a six-month educational* experience in the U.S. for "Sarah," its physical therapist who had no formal training due to its unavailability in China. Through CCPD, she enjoyed a three-month internship at Bethesda Lutheran Homes and Services, Watertown, Wisconsin, a member organization that serves people with developmental disabilities. Sarah also observed therapy techniques at four other locations in Wisconsin and Iowa. Including the time CCPD spent helping arrange for her visa, the entire process took two years.

Speaking as CCPD Director Emeritus, Joni Eareckson Tada testified in favor of the Brownback-Landrieu Bill to ban human cloning at *a Senate briefing and a White House gathering* April 10, 2002. She advocated continued research for spinal cord injury cures, but said that other cloning bills before Congress would in effect "make it a crime NOT to destroy an entire class of human beings." Government, she emphasized "must safeguard the rights of the weak and marginalized."

Following its successful Accessible Congregations Campaign, the NOD Religion and Disability Program turned its focus to *"Opening Hearts, Minds, and Doors in Seminary Communities."* Funded by the Wheat Ridge Foundation, the CCPD Executive Director helped NOD's Ginny Thornburgh organize a May 2002 meeting of representatives of 10 Lutheran seminaries (Evangelical Lutheran Church in America and

Lutheran Church-Missouri Synod). All present agreed to work toward inclusion through recruitment, curriculum, and attitudinal and architectural accessibility.

That same year, CCPD developed *guidelines for speakers* at its conferences. Based on "our vision that God allows disability to serve a purpose," the guidelines requested people-first language, recognition of the variety of Christian denominations involved in CCPD, and "please do not teach or imply that disability or sickness has resulted from lack of faith or as a judgment from God. While there may be cases where disability is the result of sin in a person's life, this is not the place to address that issue."

NEWSLETTER AND JOURNAL EQUIP MEMBERS

To equip members for advocacy and encourage participation in CCPD efforts, a newsletter was begun in October 1992. Initially it was a part of *Networks*, published by The Special Gathering, whose founder and executive director, Richard O. Stimson, was also a CCPD board member. It included CCPD news, teachers' tips, letters, a viewpoint column by Joni Tada, and issue-oriented articles on such topics as Oregon's health-care rationing plan; inclusion, choice, and dignity; counting the cost before you minister; and how James W. Fowler's "Stages of Faith" relate to people who are developmentally disabled.

Beginning in 1995, when editorial responsibilities were transferred to the CCPD office, the newsletter changed its focus to news about all types of disability ministry. A twice-yearly *Journal*, edited by David Heidemann, was developed to carry issue-oriented articles. Eventually it became a center section in each *CCPD News*. An advisory committee was established in 1996 to help gather news from the various facets of disability ministry.

For two years the Lutheran Developmental Disabilities Coalition purchased memberships for its participants and utilized one page of *CCPD News* for stories of its activities.

Because of the success of the pre-convention Christian camping conference in 2002, a "Let's Go Camping" page, written by Don Crooker, was added in the newsletter.

As a result of her story on Cordell Brown in *CCPD News*, Executive Director Marlys Taege was asked to write an expanded *article for Special Education Today magazine*. Subsequently she authored an article on environmental illness and a feature on Christian gospel singer Tony Elenburg for the same publication.

CCPD was also asked by *Mission America* to provide resources for its Celebrate Jesus 2000 outreach. CCPD recruited a resource organization in each disability ministry field for the program, and the executive director wrote an article for Mission America's *Lighthouse Movement Handbook*.

CARING CHURCH AWARDS INSTITUTED

Another important avenue of advocacy by CCPD has been its awards program. At the 1990 Congress, the Council gave its first Caring Church awards to six congregations that were exemplary in exhibiting Christ's compassion as they reached out to and with people who had disabilities. Recipients were:

Beverly Hills Baptist Church, Memphis, TN. This 300-member congregation ran a ministry to/with 100 individuals with mental disabilities who regularly attended Sunday morning, Sunday evening, and Wednesday services. The church provided buses into the city to pick up people who had no transportation.

Crossroads Christian Church, Corona, CA. Its disability ministry focused on persons who were developmentally disabled and/or deaf. The extensive program offered a choir, respite care, field trips, social events, Special Olympics, parent support group, Sunday School, outreach, and counseling.

Georgetown Christian Reformed Church, Hudsonville, MI. Its multifaceted ministry included a respite care program that matched church members with the needs of disabled individuals.

Grace Community Church, Sun Valley, CA. Over 200 volunteers ran an extensive program for persons with all types of disabilities. The church committed staff and financial resources on a large scale to reach people with special needs.

Grace Evangelical Free Church, Walworth, WI. This small church of only 40 members (70 attendees including children) spent $10,000 installing a lift in its circa 1850 sanctuary. The congregation included developmentally disabled individuals in the worship service as greeters, ushers, bulletin board keepers and as pianist. Volunteers ran vans two times on Sunday and for midweek service to pick up people. Persons with disabilities were mainstreamed in the adult Sunday School class.

Wealthy Park Baptist Church, Grand Rapids, MI. Served by a minister to the deaf, the Deaf Chapel in its education unit was said to be the longest-running deaf ministry in America. The chapel offered Sunday School and morning and evening services for deaf people, supported missionaries and held revivals to reach persons who were deaf.

As the years passed and the Caring Church awards continued, the list of recipients began to read like a "Who's Who" in Christian disability ministry. *(See Addendum for the complete list.)* Over time, most of these congregations have expanded their ministry; some unfortunately have reduced or modified their services.

At the 1990 Congress, CCPD also honored the Billy Graham Evangelistic Association for its more than 40 years of making Christ's Gospel accessible to persons with disabilities at Crusade sites. The award received publicity in the October issue of *Decision Magazine*.

CHRISTIAN CAMPS COMMENDED FOR ACCESSIBILITY

Those awards were followed with an annual recognition of a Christian camp that was uniquely accessible and inclusive. The first one, to *Spruce Lake Retreat*, Canadensis, Pennsylvania, was given at the Christian Camping International convention in November 1990.

Other recipients included *Camp Joy-El*, Greencastle, Pennsylvania (1991); *Hope Bay Bible Camp*, Pender Island, Surrey, British Columbia, Canada (1992); *WalCamp*, Kingston, Illinois (1993); *Inspiration Center*, Walworth, Wisconsin (1994); *Spring Hill Camp*, Evart, Michigan (1995); "Make Promises Happen" Program of *Central Christian Camp and Conference Center*, Guthrie, Oklahoma (1996); *White Mills Christian Camp*, White Mills, Kentucky (1997); *Meteor Ranch*, Upper Lake, California (1998); *Camp Philip*, Wautoma, Wisconsin (2000); *Westminster Woods*, Occidental, California (2001); *Camp Matz*, Watertown, Wisconsin (2002); and *Camp Echoing Hills*, Warsaw, Ohio, and *Hume Lake Christian Camp*, Fresno, California (2003).

Because so few camps met the criteria, locating camps to receive the award proved difficult, and in 1999 and 2004 no awards were given.

What did these camps do to merit the award? The following are just a few examples.

To support full participation, Spring Hill Camp added extra counselors, transportation, special housing, and adapted activities (rock climbing, advanced dramatics, cowboy camp, and ballet, jazz, and sacred dance). Many campers at Hope Bay were from the inner city, and 90% were unchurched. A number of them came to know the Lord while at camp. Meteor Ranch, a 100-acre working ranch with summer programs for people with disabilities, also established its own residential care home for six people.

Central Camp operates the nation's largest program in disability ministry. In 1995 at the time of the CCPD award, it served 1,798 persons with disabilities during 35 events on site and 7,678 at special events at other locations. It offered buddy retreats (where each child could bring a non-handicapped friend), a solo parent family retreat, grandparents/grandchild retreats, a mothers' getaway weekend, grief retreats, and family adventure days.

For over 20 years, Lutheran youth groups from throughout the country have chosen to spend a week volunteering at Camp Matz so that every camper in the various 10-week summer programs will have a non-handicapped companion during his/her stay. An unusual shallow pool with a spray fountain allows those with physical handicaps to "swim" with others.

Echoing Hills began as the vision of the Rev. D. Cordell Brown, who has overcome the many obstacles of living with cerebral palsy. Since its founding in 1967, Echoing Hills has expanded to provide residential housing at 14 facilities in the U.S.A. and has started a mission outreach to disabled people in Ghana.

AARON AWARD RECOGNIZES VOLUNTEERS

Recognizing that ministries are dependent upon volunteers who, like Aaron in the Bible, support and hold up the arms of the leaders, CCPD instituted an annual Aaron Award in 1999. Recipients include *Rich Miltner*, Columbia Station, OH, with Friendship Ministries (1999); *Nancy Malik*, Beaver Dam, WI, Special Touch Ministries (2000); *Ken Thorsen*, Rock Valley, IA, a teacher at a school for disabled students, a Special Olympics volunteer and teacher of an interdenominational Bible study for adults with mental retardation (2001); *Linda Smith*, Boston, MA, a personal care attendant for two women with cerebral palsy and director of Vision New England's disability ministry (2002); *Connie Van Roekel*, Des Moines, IA, Run and Not Grow Tired Ministry (2003); and *Don Crooker*, Modesto, CA, for his years of support to the CCPD Board (2004).

VISION AWARD HONORS INNOVATIVE LEADERSHIP

A fourth award was added in 2003 to recognize individuals who saw a need in the disability ministry community and worked compassionately, creatively and with perseverance to meet it. The first awards were given to *Robert Bursch* of Spokane, WA, and *Eleanor Prime*, Orange, CA. As chairman of the Christian Workers Conference in Washington State, Bursch instituted a Disability Track in 1992 that quickly grew to offering multiple workshops. A retired special education teacher, Prime launched a program for young adults with disabilities at the Orange County Worship Center in 1993. It included Bible study and led to the group doing a quarterly musical. Her congregation was also motivated to purchase and open a group home for adults with developmental disabilities.

The recipient in 2004 was *Ralph Bus*, Orangeville, Ontario, Canada, who, despite his physical disability, has developed awareness programs, acted as an advocate throughout Eastern Canada, and served on the Christian Reformed Church Disabilities Committee.

Through these various awards, CCPD has not only encouraged individuals, churches and organizations, but also has spotlighted and publicized creative programs and efforts.

DEVELOPING THE ORGANIZATION

After Steve Jensen completed his term as president (1991-1992), the office was moved to the Modesto, California, headquarters of Christian Berets, the ministry of the new CCPD president, Don Crooker. (Crooker served as president in 1992-1993 and again from 1999-2003. Other presidents were Cordell Brown, 1993-1995; Steve Kranz, 1995-1997; Jerry Borton, 1997-1999; and Gary Wagner, 2003-present.)

During the 1993 conference, members were asked to identify goals for CCPD. They indicated that primary importance should be placed on networking, fellowship, a clearer focus, a national office, and a funding base.

In January 1994, when Board Member Marlys Taege retired from her position with a Christian agency serving people with developmental disabilities, CCPD asked her to become its executive director on a part-time basis. The office was transferred to her home, located initially near Waukesha, Wisconsin, and on August 1, 1994, it moved with her to nearby Milwaukee. At her request, expenses were paid but she served without salary. Eventually part-time secretarial help was hired as the organization and the workload grew.

STRATEGIC PLAN ADOPTED

Recognizing the need to expand its services and achieve a more solid financial footing, the Board in 1999 developed a Strategic Plan that identified goals in six areas:

a. *Voice*–CCPD will be the voice to and for the evangelical community regarding people with disabilities.
b. *Training for members*–Provide through national and regional conferences, local chapters, and follow-up with attendees.
c. *Professionalism*–Establish the CCPD office in a business setting with a full-time executive director and office staff.
d. *Membership Growth*–Goals were established for organizational membership (250), church membership (100), and individual membership (200).
e. *Financial stability*–Institute a comprehensive development plan.
f. *Leadership development.* In conjunction with this goal, arrangements were made for CCPD members to receive discounts when attending John Maxwell Leadership Seminars.

FULL-TIME OFFICE ESTABLISHED

In 2001, a part-time paid secretary began assisting with the office workload. CCPD received a $25,000 matching grant to help facilitate the hiring of a full-time executive director and move its office to a professional location. When that grant was met, a second was approved in 2002. It too was matched within a year.

In November 2002, LisaRose Hall was hired as the first full-time, paid executive director, and her request to move the office to Indianapolis was granted. She served until July 2004, when finances required the return to a part-time position. Jim Hukill filled in on an interim basis until his appointment as executive director in October 2004, and the office was moved to Orlando, Florida, where he also heads Eleos–The Care Network, which he and his wife Rhonette founded in 1998.

Accomplishments during Hall's tenure include: (1) establishment of an Advocacy Network of people willing to pray and respond as needed/able when people with disabilities make the news; (2) making most CCPD publications available in Braille; (3) arranging for a seminary student with a disability to be mentored by multiple seasoned professionals; (4) receiving and answering numerous inquiries about housing options, the Terri Schiavo case and other disability issues; (5) expansion of the CCPD Speakers' Bureau; (6) creation of a 15th anniversary commissioned art print to encourage people to pray with/for persons with disabilities; and (7) helping Mission America plan its 2004 leadership conference.

NEW INITIATIVE: CCPD CAN

Under Hukill's leadership in 2005, CCPD embarked on a new initiative: CCPD CAN (Connecting, Advancing and Nurturing Disability Ministry). The goal is to "energize the grassroots" and make members "owners of the association." Division coordinators will be appointed for each membership category (parachurch organizations, camps, churches, and academia).

A leadership summit in 2006 will probe "Disability Ministry for the Next Decade." Because so many disability conferences are held in the Spring, the annual CCPD gathering will be moved to the Fall, beginning in October 2006 in Orlando. While restructuring in 2005, CCPD opted to encourage attendance at other disability ministry conferences rather than hold its own.

LOOKING BACK–AND FORWARD

Advocacy, education, encouragement, inspiration and networking have been the hallmarks of CCPD since its inception. From one person's idea, it grew in service and scope–supporting inclusion and accessibility, recognizing achievements, nurturing friendships, linking ministries, impacting churches, and touching lives for the Lord. Through its conferences, it provided a Christian forum for discussion and growth. Through its position papers, Christian action was encouraged in behalf of people with disabilities. Through its publications, readers were kept abreast of current disability ministry activities, accomplishments and ideas. Through its cooperation with other Christian ministries, all were enabled to do more. As its current leaders look to the future with a goal of enhanced training for organizational leaders, it is obvious that change is inevitable but the need for Christian involvement in disability ministry continues.

CCPD contact information: Christian Council on Persons with Disabilities, 4700 Millenia Boulevard, Suite 175, Orlando, FL 32839; Website: www.ccpd.org; E-mail: ccpd@ccpd.org.

ADDENDUM–CARING CHURCH AWARD RECIPIENTS

(Comments are added for only the most unusual activities.)

1990: Beverly Hills Baptist Church, Memphis, TN; Crossroads Christian Church, Corona, CA; Georgetown Christian Reformed Church, Hudsonville, MI; Grace Community Church, Sun Valley, CA; Grace Evangelical Free Church, Walworth, WI; and *Wealthy Park Baptist Church, Grand Rapids, MI.*

1991: Beth Messiah Church, Livingston, NJ (When a member developed an environmental disability [severe asthma and chemical sensitivity], the congregation created a fragrance-free atmosphere in the church building, even giving all members reminder signs for their bathroom mirrors.); College Church, Wheaton, IL; Crystal Evangelical Free Church, New Hope, MN; First Lutheran Church, Helena, MT (One-third of the 450 church members had disabilities. The church deliberately sought out and welcomed residents of group homes after their transfer to Helena when the state hospital at Boulder was depopulated. When an addition to the church was constructed, one-third of the expansion was for more space for ministry with persons who have developmental disabilities. A "sponsor" was provided for each participant in that program.); *Orland Park Reformed Church, Orland Park, IL,* and *The Special Gathering, Cocoa, FL* (Sponsored by 54 area churches, this unique ministry allowed people with developmental disabilities to have their own congregation in which they could hold most church positions, including ushers, deacons, organist and choir members. Meeting in four locations, it had a regular attendance of 175 to 200. Besides services, The Gathering sponsored picnics, plays, parties, campouts and sports teams. It also organized an advocacy group to relate to the sponsoring congregations.).

1992: Aldan Union Church, Aldan, PA; *East Side Church of God, Anderson, IN* (All church board members pledged themselves to be a caring community per 1 Corinthians 12, paying special attention to the gifts and needs of people with physical, sensory, mental, and emotional impairments.); and *Trinity Reformed Church, Rock Valley, IA.*

1993: Bethel Lutheran Church, Madison, WI; *Cathedral in the Pines* (Assembly of God), *Beaumont, TX*; *Faith Lutheran Church, Lincoln, IL*; *Trinity United Methodist Church, Lansing, MI* (Besides a variety of inclusive opportunities, this church paid for transportation to church when needed by persons with disabilities.); and *Woodland Presbyterian Church, Pineville, LA* (This congregation was cited for treating persons with disabilities "like everyone else; they participate in everything. They belong.").

1994: Walnut Creek Presbyterian Church, Walnut Creek, CA (This church was the launching pad for Congregational Awareness Ministry, which subsequently helped numerous churches start disability ministries.).

1995: First Evangelical Free Church, Fullerton, CA (Under the direction of a part-time disability ministry staff person, Individual Christian Education Plans were designed for each student in the Disabilities Ministry Program. Emotional support and crisis intervention were offered.); *Northminster Presbyterian Church, Hutchinson, KS;* and *Plymouth Heights Christian Reformed Church, Grand Rapids, MI* (A Standing Committee on Disabilities answered directly to the church council.).

1996: First Baptist Church, Hawarden, IA (This church was also a collection center for wheelchairs to be refurbished at nearby Hope Haven International Ministries.); *Big Valley Grace Church, Modesto, CA*; and *First Baptist Church, Poznan, Poland* (A pioneer in reaching out to persons with disabilities in a country where until 1989 it was illegal for persons with disabilities to be on the street.).

1997: Church of the Exceptional, Caroleen, NC (Five vans traveled a total of 250 miles each Sunday to pick up participants in this nondenominational, interracial ministry.); *McLean Bible Church, McLean, VA* (An outstanding, well-staffed ministry led to this church to sponsor an annual conference on disability ministry for other churches.); *Placentia*

Presbyterian Church, Placentia, CA (A different team cooked dinner each Wednesday for the Circle of Friendship Bible Study and fellowship activities. Caretakers were also included, and several were led to a saving faith in Christ.); and *Southeast Christian Church, Louisville, KY* (Both services were signed for the deaf; Braille song sheets were provided, and their disability ministry coordinator used a wheelchair.).

1998: Bethel Lutheran Church, Middleburg Heights, OH; Phoenix First Assembly of God, Phoenix, AZ (The church maintained nine buses with wheelchair lifts; bus routes were organized via computer. Provisions were made to accommodate people with ventilators, feeding tubes, and severe mental and physical disabilities. A disability ministry emphasis was also included in the church's annual Pastor's School, which drew 9,000 people from all over the world.); and *West Shore Evangelical Free Church, Mechanicsburg, PA.*

1999: Ascension Lutheran Church, Waukesha, WI; College Mennonite Church, Goshen, IN; and *Hope Christian Church, Tustin, CA* (Its marquee sign proclaimed "Disability Ministry Here.").

2000: St. Luke's United Methodist Church, Columbus, OH; Evangel Assembly of God, Milwaukee, WI (Sponsored a Special Touch Ministry chapter; through its ministry to over 40 nursing homes, volunteers read and provided large print Bibles for persons with visual impairments.); *First Assembly of God, Elgin, IL;* and *New Life Church, Colorado Springs, CO* (Owned 10 handicapped accessible buses that each traveled up to 60 miles every Sunday to bring nearly 150 people with disabilities for worship, education and refreshments.).

2001: Central Assembly of God, Springfield, MO; Pleasant View Mennonite Church, Goshen, IN (When a member became disabled in an accident, the church included people with disabilities on a committee that renovated his home); *Southwest Community Church, Indian Wells, CA* (an on-site medical team was provided on weekends; classroom companions accompanied children with disabilities. All greeters and parking lot attendants were instructed on meeting needs of attendees with disabilities.); and *The Special Gathering, Volusia and Indian River, FL* (A recognition of the program expansion of a previous honoree.).

2002: Bethel Temple Assembly of God, Cleburne, TX; Open Door Church, Novato, CA (Members volunteered and taught at the church's college program, the Institute for Abundant Living, for people with developmental disabilities); and *Rejoice! Lutheran Church, Omaha, NE.*

2003: Calvary Christian Reformed Church, Orange, IA; *People's Church, Fresno, CA*; *Grace Church, Eden Prairie, MN; Christ Fellowship, Palm Beach Garden, FL;* and *Zion Church, Elkhart, IN.*

2004: Cicero Christian Church, Cicero, IN; *Calvin CRC, Muskegon, MI*; *Fellowship Bible Church North, Plano, TX;* and *First Presbyterian Church, Orange, CA.*

The Friendship Ministries Story

Gwen Penning Genzink, BA

SUMMARY. This article provides a history and description of a religious organization which works with congregations to develop group worship and one-to-one mentoring relationships with people who have cognitive impairments. It tells the story of how a parent's concern for their child's special religious needs within a specific geographical area has grown to a nationwide effort at inclusion. In turn, its expansion has led to increased financial support and then to the refinement of curricula developed for its worship and mentoring approach and its outreach to seminaries. *[Article copies available for a fee from The Haworth Document Delivery Service: 1-800-HAWORTH. E-mail address: <docdelivery@haworthpress.com> Website: <http://www.HaworthPress.com> © 2006 by The Haworth Press, Inc. All rights reserved.]*

KEYWORDS. Cognitive impairments, mentoring, resources, fund raising for special programs, inclusion, seminaries

Friendship Ministries is an international, interdenominational, not-for-profit (501c3) organization whose mission is *to share God's love with people who have cognitive impairments and to enable them to become an active part of God's family.* Friendship Ministries carries out this mission by working with local churches to set up Friendship

Gwen Penning Genzink is Assistant to the Executive Director of Friendship Ministries. Before assuming this position, she served as mentor in the program for 12 years.

[Haworth co-indexing entry note]: "The Friendship Ministries Story." Penning Genzik, Gwen. Co-published simultaneously in *Journal of Religion, Disability & Health* (The Haworth Pastoral Press, an imprint of The Haworth Press, Inc.) Vol. 10, No. 1/2, 2006, pp. 163-170; and: *Disability Advocacy Among Religious Organizations: Histories and Reflections* (ed: Albert A. Herzog, Jr.) The Haworth Pastoral Press, an imprint of The Haworth Press, Inc., 2006, pp. 163-170. Single or multiple copies of this article are available for a fee from The Haworth Document Delivery Service [1-800-HAWORTH, 9:00 a.m. - 5:00 p.m. (EST). E-mail address: docdelivery@ haworthpress.com].

doi:10.1300/J095v10n01_11

groups, which center on group worship and one-to-one Bible study in the context of mentoring relationships. Beyond assisting churches in initiating and maintaining Friendship programs, Friendship Ministries advocates for the inclusion of people with cognitive impairments in the full life of their faith communities, encouraging full church membership and opportunities for people with cognitive impairments to share their gifts.

Friendship Ministries got its start in 1979 when Jack and Dorothy Wiersma, parents of Sherman, who has Down syndrome, approached CRC Publications, the publishing division of their denomination, the Christian Reformed Church. They asked what Sunday school materials were available that would be appropriate for their son, and the answer was "none." Realizing that the need for such materials was great, CRC Publications, under the leadership of James Heynen, moved quickly to address the need, searching out a model for the program and hiring an editor to develop study materials.

A model group, found at Third Reformed Church in Holland, Michigan, embodied what would become the defining characteristics of Friendship groups: the group met first for fellowship, worship, prayer, and a lesson, followed by a time in which students and teachers broke off into one-to-one time to personalize and reinforce the lesson and to form relationships.

The Third Reformed Church group had also begun at the impetus of a parent: the late John Brinkman, father of a son with cognitive impairments, approached Professor Garret Wilterdink of Western Theological Seminary in Holland with the need for the church to minister to youth and adults with cognitive impairments. Professor Wilterdink then suggested to seminary student Bill Paarlberg that he create such a program for his master's thesis. He did so by establishing the mentoring model and creating study materials, and the group first met at Third Reformed Church in the fall of 1969 with six students and six teachers. Mr. Paarlberg led the group and told the story, while the late Marcy Vanderwel, a local special education teacher, led the group singing.

The program grew rapidly as word spread through local parent networks, and in the fall of 1970 the group divided to provide one section for youth (those younger than high school age) and one for adults (those of high school age or older). Martie Bultman joined the ministry at this time as leader of the adult level, and when Bill Paarlberg graduated from seminary the following year and moved on, Marcy Vanderwel took responsibility for the youth level.

From the beginning Third Reformed Church's ministry was guided by a board of directors, made up mostly of parents, and was supported financially by local groups from the Reformed Church in America and the Christian Reformed Church. Participants were recruited each fall through newspaper articles on the Saturday religion page of the local paper, through announcements in local church bulletins, and through contacts at Hope College in Holland and at Western Theological Seminary. Critical support also came from Don and Elsa van Reken, parents of one of the students in the group, who typed and copied the study materials created by Mr. Paarlberg.

Having seen in the Third Reformed Church group an inspiring model of what ministry with people who have cognitive impairments could become, CRC Publications undertook the project of developing curricula to be used by such groups. Under the direction of editor Pat Nederveld, who had experience in special education, the publications staff developed a Scripture plan for the materials and recruited Marcy Vanderwel and Martie Bultman to write the curriculum based on their existing ministry model. The first materials, consisting of three years of curriculum titled *Year One: God Our Father*, *Year Two: Jesus Our Savior*, and *Year Three: The Spirit Our Helper* were published in 1982. To ensure the excellence of these materials, the publisher submitted them for the review of numerous experts, including staff members at the Christian Learning Center in Grand Rapids, Michigan.

It quickly became apparent that the materials needed to be promoted and supported by a ministry separate from CRC Publications. The Friendship Foundation was organized in 1982 as an interdenominational ministry governed by a board of directors, many of whom ended up serving for nearly fourteen years. Cele Mereness, who had experience establishing and promoting several Sunday school programs, served as Friendship's first director. The early vision that Friendship would be interdenominational was a critical direction-setting decision that is responsible for Friendship's current scope. Over the past twenty or so years Friendship has worked with churches and organizations in more than forty denominations in twenty-some countries in North and South America, Australia, Africa, and Asia.

Other critical philosophical elements were also in place from the beginning. The overarching goal of the program was that people with cognitive impairments and their families would experience God's love for them through the embrace of the church. For younger children with cognitive impairments, this would mean finding ways to include them in regular Sunday school activities with their peers. When this inclusion began to fall apart, often in the early teenage years, the Friendship program would step in to ensure that the church was nurturing the faith of these older children and adults in ways that would be meaningful to them. Friendship programs were not meant to substitute for inclusion in the rest of the church; on the contrary, they were to supplement involvement in the church with a place where people with cognitive impairments could both explore their faith and form relationships.

Early promotion of the Friendship program was done on a very small budget and mainly in Christian Reformed congregations in the United States and Canada, as this was the group in which the earliest networking opportunities existed. Expansion into other denominations took place by the word-of-mouth, grassroots efforts of many people, most visibly parents of children with cognitive impairments, as well as through some small church conferences. Church education leaders proved to be important gatekeepers in the local churches; numerous phone calls were made to them, and sample packs of materials were distributed.

Most churches were quick to see the need for ministry with people with cognitive impairments; one hurdle, however, was–and still is–finding people within the church to run with the program. Early leaders were often parents and special education teachers. But Friendship Ministries staff encouraged the idea that anyone can be a Friendship leader, and they especially addressed senior citizens with this message. The key was simply getting people to give it a try. Mentors quickly discover how important this ministry is and that the relationships are not one-way teaching relationships; instead they are friendships in which each friend has something to offer and something to gain.

One need that became apparent early on was a resource to facilitate the process of helping people with cognitive impairments become full members of their congregations, whether through baptism, confirmation, or profession of faith. In response to this need, Friendship Ministries worked with chaplain and author Rev. Ronald Vredeveld to produce a book called *Expressing Faith in Jesus*. This resource is now in its third edition, which includes an accompanying resource kit and an emphasis on opportunities for all members of the body of Christ to use their gifts in the church.

During the 1980s a significant endowment fund was established through the generosity of longtime board member Elsa Prince and her husband, the late Edward Prince. The endowment has allowed Friendship Ministries to contribute grants to CRC Publications–now called Faith Alive Christian Resources, which continues to publish Friendship materials–for the design, development, and editing of new materials, making possible the publication of resources that are often not financially self-supporting.

In 1986 Friendship Groups Canada was established as a separate charity with its own board of directors and staff. The focus of this organization is to begin and nurture Friendship groups in Canada. The current executive director, Meta Shamrock, is based in Kitchener, Ontario.

Additional study resources were developed in the 1990s, including *Living God's Way*, a course on the Ten Commandments, developed by the leaders of a Friendship group in Calgary, Alberta. This was followed by ten *Life Studies*, short courses on thematic topics such as "When People Die," "Growing Closer to God," and "We All Have Gifts." These *Life Studies*, which were originally designed for use by higher-functioning friends, were subsequently supplemented with alternative activities to reach a broader range of students present in most groups by a grant of $25,000 from the W.K. Kellogg Foundation, which also funded the development of *Caring Relationships*, a resource that addresses sexuality and people with cognitive impairments. Other grants have also supported Friendship Ministries' publishing and operating expenses over the years.

Friendship's reach across the United States was aided by a network of area representatives initiated in 1994. Area representatives attended local church conferences and worked with local churches to establish Friendship groups, offering the kind of intensive follow-up that can be difficult from a distance. They also attended yearly meetings held by Friendship Ministries. Though the area representative approach was formally phased out in 2003, several representatives continue to work in their local areas in coordination with Friendship staff.

A highlight for the spread of the Friendship Ministries vision occurred in 1996 when Director Cele Mereness spent three weeks in Australia and one week in New Zealand. The trip, organized by Joanne Van Waginengen of Mt. Evelyn, Victoria, Australia, included numerous media contacts as well as meetings with local churches out of which several Friendship groups began. Cele Mereness retired the following year, at which time Nella Uitvlugt became executive director, bringing to the position professional experience in special education. In 1997 there was also a name change from "Friendship Foundation" to "Friendship Ministries," as well as a new logo.

At the same time translation of *Year Two: Jesus Our Savior* into Spanish began. Elizabeth Rodriguez Waterfield became the representative for Friendship's Spanish-language ministry, *Ministerio Amistad*, in 2002. Today there are approximately sixty *Amistad* groups in fifteen countries, primarily in North and South America. *Ministerio Amistad* has spread through grassroots efforts, presence at conferences, and advertising in magazines such as *Alcanzando los niños*, a magazine for people working with at-risk children. Financial support to provide materials for groups that cannot afford them has been raised through a special *Amistad* fund. Translation of *Year One: God Our Father* into Spanish is currently under way.

In January of 1999 the Friendship Ministries Board of Directors spent a day on strategic planning. Several key decisions were made, including the rewriting of Friendship's mission and vision statements and initiation of a revision of its aging study materials. These revisions were undertaken with a firm commitment to produce high-quality materials, and more than thirty people, many with special education backgrounds, were involved in the process. The revisions included expanding the range of activities suggested in the Bible Studies to address the needs of a wider variety of learners, as well as a focus on creating full color visuals that communicate clearly and consistently. It also involved wording changes that reflect Friendship's commitment to inclusivity and affirmation of the fact that relationships are never one-way. Thus the materials no longer refer to "students" and "teachers," but rather to "friends" and "mentors." Revision of the three series *God Our Father, Jesus Our Savior*, and *The Spirit Our Helper* (now referred to as *Friendship Bible Studies*) was completed in 2005.

A document created in 2002 titled "First Things" further identified biblical principals that both motivate and shape the work of Friendship Ministries. It outlines foundational themes that guide decision-making by the Board of Directors, as well as core truths that guide communication of Friendship Ministries' mission and its theological and philosophical roots. Two other important documents, the "Friendship Ministries Model Guidelines' for Abuse Prevention" and the "Friendship Program Model Volunteer Disclosure Form," were adopted in 2004 for the protection of all members of Friendship groups.

The curriculum revision project required Friendship Ministries' largest fundraising effort to date, spearheaded by board member Ralph Honderd. His work was so successful that within six weeks the goal was nearly reached. The goal was eventually exceeded, allowing for expansion of the project to include additional materials such as separate Christmas and Easter books, as well as CDs containing music for the songs included in the Bible Studies.

Fundraising necessarily involved raising awareness among donors, and Ralph Honderd and his wife, Carol, eventually expanded their role as volunteers to include traveling across the United States to raise awareness in local churches and seminaries. Their grassroots work has been critical to starting new groups and supporting existing ones. To date they have visited fourteen seminaries, encouraging them to include a disability awareness component in their courses of study.

Friendship Ministries has worked particularly closely with two seminaries, Calvin Theological Seminary in Grand Rapids, MI and Western Theological Seminary in Holland, MI, to create tools describing their efforts to address disability concerns for use by other seminaries. Western Theological Seminary has also taken on a groundbreaking residential project that will have people with cognitive impairments living side-by-side with seminary students and sharing fellowship together. The project has been called "Friendship House" in recognition of the work of Friendship Ministries.

Research undertaken for Friendship Ministries by The Greystone Group in 2004 indicates that participants in Friendship groups exhibit a passion and conviction not seen in many other ministries, and that observable changes in participants, volunteers, and congregations involved in Friendship Ministries are more evident than in many ministries. With this potential for positive change in mind, Friendship Ministries has embraced the importance of thinking of itself not simply as a curriculum provider but as a ministry that holistically addresses the spiritual needs of people with cognitive impairments and their churches. In addition to the research done by The Greystone Group, Friendship has recently undertaken a research project with Joan Bacon, Professor of Education at Augustana College in Sioux Falls, South Dakota. This research will examine the changing attitudes of seminarians through their involvement in Friendship groups. Jeff McNair, Education Professor at California Baptist University, is also researching the changes that take place in a church that has a Friendship program.

Meanwhile, work is progressing on a book on Pervasive Developmental Disorders/Autism Spectrum Disorders (PDD/ASD) and spirituality aimed to help churches address the spiritual needs of people with PDD/ASD and to include them in the church. Though Friendship programs are not an ideal fit for all individuals with PDD/ASD, some have been part of Friendship programs for many years and have thrived there. The book also includes strategies for use in Friendship programs, in churches, and in inclusive Christian schools.

Friendship Ministries has developed key relationships through membership in the Christian Council on Persons with Disabilities, with whom Friendship has cosponsored a number of conferences, the American Association on Mental Retardation's Religion and Spirituality Division, and the National Apostolate for Inclusion Ministries. Friendship also regularly attends conferences of the National Catholic Partnership on Disability, the National Council of Churches in Christ's Education Committee on Disabilities, the National Down Syndrome Society, and the National Down Syndrome Congress, among others. Contacts with local care providers and local ARC chapters have been key grassroots methods of connecting people with local resources to address spiritual needs. Developing relationships with the Christian Learning Center and with singer/songwriter Ken Medema provide additional opportunities to increase awareness and to strengthen ministry with people who have cognitive impairments.

Looking to the future, Friendship Ministries is excited about opportunities to help make churches not only accessible but also inclusive. In addition to helping churches start and nurture Friendship groups, Friendship Ministries' extensive consulting efforts will continue to encourage Disability Awareness Sundays and to share ideas on including children with disabilities in regular Sunday school, offering a spiritual IEP (Individualized Education Program) tool as an important resource. They will also emphasize the importance of full church membership and opportunities for people with cognitive impairments to share their gifts within the church. Mentors will be encouraged to become even more involved in the lives of their friends, getting to know them as whole persons and advocating for them at Person-Centered Planning meetings.

Partnerships will continue to be crucial for accomplishing these goals. As a cosponsor of the historic Interfaith Disability Pre-Summit to the Alliance for Full Participation held this past September, Friendship Ministries has a vision for what can be accomplished as we increase dialogue between secular and faith-based organizations. Friendship Ministries also sees international opportunities to support service providers with templates for creating materials and services that promote spiritual growth and inclusion in churches around the world. In all its efforts, Friendship Ministries will continue to reach across denominational lines to share God's love with people who have cognitive impairments and to enable them to be an active part of God's family.

Joni and Friends:
From a Founder's Heart
to a Fledgling Worldwide
Disability Missions Ministry

Pastor Dan'l C. Markham

SUMMARY. This paper documents the history of *Joni and Friends* as a worldwide missions ministry to people with disabilities which, in 2005, celebrated its 25th anniversary. The organization's ministry, while initially an outgrowth of one person's struggle with a disability (Joni Eareckson Tada), developed into a worldwide ministry of witness and service in which evangelical witness was deemed as important as providing wheelchairs to the persons needing them. Gradually, the ministry has grown to a point where ministries in the United States and around the globe function independently yet in a highly integrated manner with the Joni and Friends International Disability Center. Especially significant is its focus on the needs of people with disabilities in developing and formerly communist nations. *[Article copies available for a fee from The Haworth Document Delivery Service: 1-800-HAWORTH. E-mail address: <docdelivery@haworthpress. com> Website: <http://www.HaworthPress.com> © 2006 by The Haworth Press, Inc. All rights reserved.]*

Pastor Dan'l C. Markham, Director of Field Operations for *Joni and Friends*, has devoted most of his professional life developing Christian minorities, programs, and projects, possessing a passion to minister and mobilize ministry to the marginalized.

[Haworth co-indexing entry note]: "*Joni and Friends*: From a Founder's Heart to a Fledgling Worldwide Disability Missions Ministry." Markham, Dan'l C. Co-published simultaneously in *Journal of Religion, Disability & Health* (The Haworth Pastoral Press, an imprint of The Haworth Press, Inc.) Vol. 10, No. 1/2, 2006, pp. 171-194; and: *Disability Advocacy Among Religious Organizations: Histories and Reflections* (ed: Albert A. Herzog, Jr.) The Haworth Pastoral Press, an imprint of The Haworth Press, Inc., 2006, pp. 171-194. Single or multiple copies of this article are available for a fee from The Haworth Document Delivery Service [1-800-HAWORTH, 9:00 a.m. - 5:00 p.m. (EST). E-mail address: docdelivery@haworthpress.com].

Available online at http://www.haworthpress.com/web/JRDH
© 2006 by The Haworth Press, Inc. All rights reserved.
doi:10.1300/J095v10n01_12

KEYWORDS. *Joni and Friends*, Joni Eareckson Tada, disability in developing countries, disability in former communist countries, Europe, Africa, Asia, Wheels for the World

INTRODUCTION

The history of *Joni and Friends* as a fledgling worldwide missions ministry is at its core the study of the seeds of God's Word sown in the heart of a child, nurtured in the heart of a teenager, and forged like steel in the furnace of suffering in the life of a young woman struggling with the emotional, spiritual, and physical effects of quadriplegia. It is the study of the growth of a child of God into a woman of God (Joni Eareckson Tada), now a world-renowned Christian personality, acquaintance of presidents, kings, prime ministers, and paupers alike. More important, many would contend, she is the beloved spokesperson and spiritual magnet of millions of people affected by disability[1] who make up a hidden people group of 650 million people worldwide–about 10 percent of the world's population.[2]

This then is the study of these seeds grown in this heart and, in turn, grafted into the hearts of scores, then hundreds, then thousands, and now millions of people around the world, fostering not only a world-class parachurch ministry, *Joni and Friends*, but the woman and, increasingly more so, the ministry providing leadership for a worldwide movement in response to the Luke 14:12-24 mandate of Christ: "Go out quickly into the streets and alleys of the town and bring in the poor, the crippled, the blind, and the lame . . . make them come in, so that my house will be full" (vs. 21, 23, NIV).[3]

A WORLDWIDE NEED

In 1996 the World Health Organization put the number of people with disability at "up to 600 million."[4] There is a need, especially in developing countries, for over 20 million wheelchairs.[5]

Disabled people around the world live in unbelievable poverty and isolation, lacking simple mobility and cut off from society and from the Gospel of Jesus Christ. Of these 600-650 million people, it is believed that in majority countries somewhere in the vicinity of only 5-10 percent are effectively reached with the Gospel (*Joni and Friends'* anecdotal conversations and internal reports), arguably making the disability community one of the largest unreached–some say under-reached–or hidden people groups in the world. Jesus surely made them a target group of the Great Commission (compare Luke 14:12-24 to Matthew 18:18-20).[6]

There are approximately 54 million people, or 20.6 percent of the U.S. population, who have a disability; and of this group, 26 million Americans have a severe disability.[7] This higher percentage in the U.S. compared to majority countries is thought to be attributable to better medical services and thus higher survival rates and longevity.

Information from the 1998 National Health Survey shows that 26 percent of U.S. adults who seek pastoral care from a priest, minister, rabbi, or other religious counselor have disabilities. The percent increases with age and is higher among women–52 percent. People with disabilities are more than twice as likely as persons without disabilities to seek pastoral care: 8.1 percent disabled compared to 4 percent able-bodied.[8] Just in the United States the unemployment rate amongst the disabled is 63 percent. Over 80 percent of families with a disabled member experience divorce. Abuse, alienation, and depression are common in this segment of the population.[9]

Dr. Michael Beates, Board Member of *Joni and Friends*, explained in his doctoral thesis for Reformed Theological Seminary:

> People with disabilities are nearly universally absent from the congregations of America's churches. In 1 Corinthians 12: 14-27 the Apostle Paul describes the church using the metaphor of the human body. He said that "God has arranged the parts of the body, every one of them, just as he wanted them to be" (v. 18). Some he describes as weaker but indispensable and others as less honorable and less respectable but treated with special honor and greater respect (vv. 22-23). Certainly on one level Paul is describing people with disabilities, broken people as part of Christ's body, the new community. And his description of the Christian community should be understood as normative.
>
> Statistics from many sources number Americans with disabilities at over 40 million people. This is approximately one in every six citizens. But even a casual survey of most American congregations shows that these 'weaker, indispensable, and especially honorable members' are, for the most part, simply not there. They certainly are not represented proportional to their numbers in the national population. Nearly twenty years ago (long before the

Americans With Disabilities Act), Joni Eareckson Tada wrote, "Ten percent of our population is severely disabled. (That's a flat figure, including impairments of all sorts.) So theoretically, on any given Sunday, a pastor ought to look out over his people and see ten percent who are limited–the deaf, the blind, people in wheelchairs–whatever."

Such people have not been purposely excluded, and most church members and leaders would certainly affirm that people with disabilities are welcome at their particular church. But those who live with disabilities (that is, those who are disabled, and those who live with and care for someone who is disabled) will testify that, though American culture generally is becoming more aware of and responsive to the needs and abilities of this disabled segment of society (especially since the Americans With Disabilities Act in 1990), in many subtle ways people with disabilities sense a lack of welcome from the church. Nancy Eiseland agrees, writing, "The history of the church's interaction with the disabled is at best an ambiguous one. Rather than being a structure for empowerment, the church has more often supported the societal structures and attitudes that have treated people with disabilities as objects of pity and paternalism. For many disabled persons the church has been a 'city on a hill'–physically inaccessible and socially inhospitable."[10]

These needs and challenges faced by the disabled in the developing world are compounded by even greater ignorance, prejudice, and lack of a Christian worldview towards the marginalized. Joni Eareckson Tada wrote:

However, there are factors other than physical needs which must also be considered. The handicapping conditions of discrimination, fear, and pity imposed by other people must be removed. Disabled people have had to learn to play the part of the cowering and indebted in order to survive in the world of the physically capable. They are often treated as if they are children. These unjust social handicaps keep disabled people locked in dependency and poverty.

This is the real message behind Luke 14:12-14. The parable has less to do with "lending a hand to those helpless invalids," and more to do with landing a knockout blow to the religious and social hierarchy which perpetuated the institutionalized discrimination against disabled people.[11]

A BIBLICAL MANDATE TO THE WHOLE WORLD INCLUDING THOSE WITH DISABILITIES

According to Doug Mazza, President of *Joni and Friends*, *Joni and Friends* views its mission statement–"To communicate the Gospel and equip Christ-honoring churches worldwide to evangelize and disciple people affected by disability"–as being based upon what it contends is a biblical mandate capsulated in Luke 14:12-24, the text including the Parable of the Great Banquet Feast.[12] It would be hard to argue against the contention that today *Joni and Friends* is nothing less than a worldwide ministry with worldwide evangelism and missions being its very heartbeat–its heartbeat realized and lived out through the organization's mission statement.

Celebrating its 25th anniversary in January 2004, *Joni and Friends* paused to reflect upon and summarize the state of the ministry nationally and internationally:

- Communications

    - Radio. Twenty-two years of broadcasting and over 5,600 recorded daily programs later, *Joni and Friends* is presently "heard on over 1,000 radio outlets by an estimated one million listeners per week."[13] Additionally, this involves rebroadcasts internationally via the *Joni and Friends* website (www.joniandfriends.org) and through foreign stations.
    - Print Media. Over 30 books authored by Joni Eareckson Tada, translated into over 45 languages, distributed in over 50 countries. In May 2004, Zondervan Publishing noted on its website (*www.zondervan.com/Books/Detail.asp*) that the 25th Anniversary edition of Joni's most popular book, her autobiography *Joni*, has more than 3,000,000 copies in print in over 40 languages. Articles every year are published in national and international periodicals about Joni, *Joni and Friends*, *Wheels for the World*, and the ministry's other initiatives.

- Television. Numerous appearances on secular and religious programs.
- Movie. The World Wide Pictures feature film production *Joni*, released in 1979, has been translated into 14 languages and has been viewed by at least 40 million people.[14]
- Speaking engagements by Joni Eareckson Tada, President Doug Mazza, and other staff members to scores of churches, conferences, missions groups, and international disability, religious, and mission convocations.

- *Wheels for the World* (WFTW), in cooperation with U.S. Field Offices (Satellite offices and Area Ministries), mobilize and train WFTW outreach teams (short-term missionaries/STMs) who conduct wheelchair distributions in conjunction with evangelism efforts in numerous countries each year.

    - WFTW conducts disability ministry training seminars to equip nationals, indigenous churches, and parachurch ministries to grow effective and culturally appropriate disability ministries.
    - In 2004, 5,477 were distributed to a minimum of 12 countries via 13 outreaches involving STMs from scores of churches.[15] This will involve close to 1,000 volunteers, 7 corporate sponsors, 11 U.S. prisons and one Polish prison where donated used wheelchairs are restored.[16] WFTW has impacted over 2,000,000 people in the last ten years.[17]
    - Every person receiving a wheelchair is personally fitted to his/her chair. They and their family receive Gospel literature and Bibles, and usually hear a presentation of the salvation message. This often involves outreach by our foreign church partners, who usually have evangelistic services in conjunction with a wheelchair distribution.
    - WFTW Harvest Project encourages churches and parachurch ministries to expand their missions program to people affected by disability by forming an alliance with the *Wheels for the World* international outreach. "*Wheels for the World* will 'sow seed' by providing wheelchairs and other disability equipment for your outreach to a developing country. Reaping takes place as your church or parachurch ministry provides the gift of mobility and God's saving grace . . . unto the least of these."[18]

- Foreign Chartered and Affiliate Partners (19) in Albania, Ghana, India, Isle of Man, The Netherlands, New Zealand, Peru, Poland, Portugal, Romania, Togo, and United Kingdom.

  - Charters and Affiliates train and conduct their own disability intercultural and cross-cultural outreaches. They are staffed by nationals and are self-funded. For example, the India Affiliate, Beulah Ministries, reaches seven different language groups in India as well as equipping and sending church planting and evangelism teams to nearby Pakistan, Nepal, and Bangladesh. The Poland Charter, staffed by nationals and completely Polish supported, conducts outreaches to Ukraine.
  - Additionally, WFTW partners with other international ministries that conduct missionary work in foreign countries, such as Josh McDowell Ministries, Operation Chair Lift, Global Transformation, Equip India, and *It Is Written*.

- U.S.-based Ministry Affiliates. Affiliates such as Child Evangelism Fellowship (CEF), Mission to Unreached Peoples, and Global Transformation receive training, printed resources, and sometimes funding from *Joni and Friends*.
- Strategic Partnerships. From its inception *Joni and Friends* has partnered on the foreign field at the program and project level with a number of national and international ministries such as the Billy Graham Evangelistic Association. In the winter of 2003-4, *Joni and Friends* and Reformed Theological Seminary (RTS), Virtual Campus Charlotte, North Carolina, launched a training initiative providing ministry training worldwide as part of ongoing partnership envisioned to provide evangelical theological training and practical disability ministry skills. *Joni and Friends* sees itself as a storefront for RTS to reach the disabled and others called to the disability community for training in the U.S. and around the world. As part of this partnership, Reformed Theological Seminary and *Joni and Friends* offer a 15-credit Disability Ministry Certificate.
- Ministry Associates. Ministries Associates (Christian workers, missionaries, and ordained ministers with a specific call to the disability community) conduct evangelism, discipleship, and help ministries nationally and internationally in partnership with *Joni and Friends*.

- The Christian Fund for the Disabled (CFD). A small grants program available to churches, parachurch organizations, missionary organizations, and individuals affected by disabilities in the U.S. and around the world, CFD has funded such efforts as disability ministry training seminars, evangelistic endeavors, micro-enterprise efforts, theological training for people affected by disabilities, and projects to make churches accessible to the disabled.
- *On A Roll for Jesus*! (OAR4J) Vacation Bible School missions curriculum. According to *Joni and Friends* Marketing Manager Cheri Van Houten, the fruit of this three-year-old program has resulted in "involving over 60,000 children who raised some $375,000, resulting in 2,500 wheelchairs being restored and shipped to foreign countries with Gospel bracelets and Gospel literature."
- Prayer and Worship. Foundational in the life of Joni and in the ministry of *Joni and Friends* is prayer and worship.[19] Furthermore, Joni Eareckson Tada sees the ministry of prayer related to evangelism and world missions having special application to the disabled who have restricted mobility,[20] calling attention to her story about a quadriplegic friend, Diane:

> Every morning Connie opens Diane's bedroom door to begin the long routine of exercising and bathing her severely paralyzed friend. The story is the same each dawn of every new day at Connie and Diane's apartment. The routine rarely changes. Sunrise stretches into mid-morning by the time Diane is ready to sit up in her wheelchair. But those long hours in bed are significant.
>
> In her quiet sanctuary, Diane turns her head slightly on the pillow toward the corkboard on the wall. Her eyes can scan each thumbtacked card and list. Each photo, every torn piece of paper carefully pinned in a row. This stillness is broken as Diane begins to murmur.
>
> She is praying. . . . Diane is confident, convinced her life is significant. Her labor of prayer counts. She moves mountains that block the paths of missionaries. She helps open the eyes of the spiritually blind in Southeast Asia. She pushes back the kingdom of darkness that blackens the alleys and streets of the gangs in East L.A.

Diane is on the front lines, advancing the Gospel of Christ, holding up weak saints, inspiring doubting believers, energizing other prayer warriors, and delighting her Lord and Savior.[21]

FROM A FOUNDER'S HEART TO A WORLDWIDE MINISTRY

The growth and development of *Joni and Friends* into a worldwide missions ministry has been an unfolding revelation of God's will and God's Word in tandem with God's provision and direction in the life of Joni Eareckson Tada and in those God has brought around her as the *Joni and Friends* team, now some 75 employees, a thousand volunteers or more per year, and thousands of donors. This history can be seen in seven fairly distinct phases:

- The Formative Years (1949-1966)
- The Defining Moment and Years of Struggle (1967-1973)
- The Ministry Launching Years (1974-1982)
- The Ministry Learning Years (1983-1989)
- The Building Years (1990-1998)
- The Transition Years (1999-2003)
- The Capstone Year (2003-4)
- The Years to Come (2004-)

The Formative Years (1949-1966)

Many say the story begins at the time of a diving accident. "Her own story began on a hot July afternoon in 1967. Tada dove into a shallow lake and suffered a spinal cord fracture that left her paralyzed from the neck down."[22] But in reality, the story–i.e., history of missions of *Joni and Friends* as spiritual seeds sown, germinated, and birthed in Joni Eareckson's heart–started much earlier. In an interview (March 8, 2004) Joni revealed the formative elements in her heart and mind that provided fertile ground for a missions-driven heart. These were provided by her family's strong biblical faith, fall mission conferences at her evangelical church, and a trip to Cuba when she was five-years-old during which she was deeply impacted observing people in the grips of poverty.[23]

Perhaps the most formative ingredients were to be works of the Holy Spirit in Joni Eareckson's heart. While raised in a family of faith and an evangelical environment, Joni had yet to have a personal encounter with the Lord she and her family served and worshipped. But that would change when this 14-year-old girl attended a Young Life meeting in Natural Bridge, Virginia. She writes, " . . . I felt my heart open to the Gospel being presented by our Young Life speaker. When he asked if any of us wanted to pray to embrace Christ as Savior, I readily responded. That evening I found myself back at the camp meeting hall. . . . I noticed during the meeting that everything looked and felt different. . . . Before, the hymns and Gospel songs were fun to sing, but now they *meant* something."[24]

While God continued to work in the heart of Joni in the following three years, it was in that third year following her conversion experience, at the age of 17, as she struggled with normal teenage temptations, she reveals a specific preparatory work of the Holy Spirit just days before the most defining moment of her life (her diving accident). "I thought back to my prayer earlier in the year: 'God, do something, *anything*, in my life to change me.' I was convinced God was about to alter my life. I just didn't know what he would do or where, when, or how it would happen. If my ears could have tuned in, I might have picked up the signal. I might have heard God whispering, 'I have something in mind for you. Something above the norm. Can you trust me? Can you follow me?'"[25]

The Defining Moment and Years of Struggle (1967-1973)

It could be said that the seed that eventually became a full grown tree of a worldwide ministry–*Joni and Friends*–was germinated, was given life at the very point of the death of Joni Eareckson's more-than-promising life as a stellar athlete and student. Some would say that dive into the shallow waters of Chesapeake Bay in July of 1967 was a fateful day; yet today Joni would say, and does say, it was a day of God's sovereign working. Many tortuous, even terrifying, days would follow, and those days were, in turn, followed with years of struggle regarding her faith, wrestling with stark and painful yet profound theological questions as to God's will, sovereignty, and purposes in her life.

Nonetheless, the defining moment of her life was that day in which the "God she loves" implemented His divine purposes through a life-shattering shallow dive. Interestingly, as she reveals in her most recent book, her memoir *The God I Love*, her final thought before that dive was about the goodness of God. "Waves slapped the side of the raft and sparkled like diamonds. Yes, I was glad I'd come. To feel my body, to be blonde and tanned, fit, and looking forward to college. *God is good*, I thought, summing it up. I smoothed my bathing suit, then stretched my arms above my head, arched my back, and jibed offhandedly to the boys, 'Watch this,' planning to show them a simple inward-pike dive. And I dove for the keel."

While the year 1974 marked the beginning of a national public ministry for Joni with her appearance on the *Today Show* with Barbara Walters, it was during the previous six years that Joni was formed into a one-of-a-kind servant of Christ. These were crucible years of Christ-character forming and theological forming and foundations. While the official incorporation of *Joni and Friends* occurred in 1979, in a spiritual sense these were the years (1967-1973) that *Joni and Friends* as a worldwide missionary ministry was created–created in the heart and mind of a young, bright, quadriplegic Christian, struggling with issues of faith and the heart and mind of God.

Joni has had some excellent mentors along the way, including her husband Ken Tada, Pastor Charles Swindoll, Dr. Billy Graham, and Pastor John MacArthur, but no one person has been as instrumental in her life, from a biblical or theological point of view, as her life-long friend, Steve Estes. Steve, who holds Master of Divinity and Master of Theology degrees and is pastor of Community Evangelical Free Church in Elverson, Pennsylvania, tells of the first encounter with Joni. He was then a 16-year-old student of the Bible, and she the good looking, bright, popular 19-year-old quadriplegic loaded with some serious biblical and theological questions. After no more than ten minutes of her first encounter with Steve, Joni challenged him, "So, Diana says you're big into the Bible. Tell me, do you think God had anything to do with my breaking my neck?"[26]

He recorded his answer to Joni's direct and probing question. This answer matured in subsequent years of joint Bible study into a system of theology on suffering, which was capsulated in their co-authored book, *When God Weeps*. His first answer, brave but not brash, proved to be the foundation of Joni's theological make up: "God put you in that chair, Joni. I don't know why, but if you'll trust him instead of fighting him, you'll find out why–if not in this life, then in the next. He let you break your neck because he loves you."[27]

As the next four years ticked away, Joni not only wrestled with God and came to terms with her life as it was, and to terms with God as she came to understand Him, she began to blossom as a local Christian public speaker and somewhat locally celebrated mouth artist. God's purposes were beginning to come into reality for her.

The Ministry Launching Years (1974-1981)

It was her art that would launch her into the public's consciousness. Shortly after appearing in 1974 on a local television news show that featured her as a mouth artist, she found herself on the *Today Show* with Barbara Walters. From there Joni's life began to accelerate in Christian ministry. A publisher, seeing her on the *Today Show*, offered her a book deal, which resulted in her best-selling autobiography *Joni*, first published in 1976. That same year she was a speaking guest at a nationally televised Billy Graham Crusade. In 1979 the movie *Joni* (World Wide Pictures), starring Joni Eareckson, premiered with considerable success. Also in 1979, with the counsel and support of the Billy Graham Evangelistic Association, the ministry *Joni and Friends* was incorporated and launched, beginning in a modest office in Burbank, California.

In 1978 Joni's first major writing project with Steve Estes, *A Step Further*, was published, launching Joni's role as a highly regarded teacher on disability ministry. This, her second book with Zondervan publishing, cemented what would become a long-term relationship with the publishing company.

The Ministry Learning Years (1982-1989)

Eight events broadened the vision of Joni and *Joni and Friends* and moved the ministry into the international arena, providing formative thought, prayer, planning, and action regarding the arena of world missions:

- The *Joni and Friends* radio program was launched (1982).
- *Joni and Friends* begins the Joy in Caring Seminar, which was held in 17 U.S. cities (1982-88).
- A ministry trip to Romania (1982).
- The Christian Fund for the Disabled matching grant program was initiated (1987).
- The first-ever Congress on the Church and Disability convened (1988).
- Joni is founding president of the Christian Council on Persons with Disabilities (1988).

- Joni gave the keynote presentation on disability ministry at the Lausanne Conference on World Evangelization in Manila (1989).
- Joni spoke at the Billy Graham Association's crusade in Hungary, seeing "hundreds, maybe thousands, of disabled people (were) hobbling into the giant stadium."[28] At the close of the opening night of the crusade, 35,000 people came forward to receive Christ.

From 1982-1989 the needs of the church were identified and clarified in regards to reaching those affected by disabilities, when detailed and comprehensive concepts of disability ministry were discovered and developed, resulting in such practical *Joni and Friends* publications as *How To Create An Effective Disability Ministry in Your Church* (now titled *Through The Roof*), by Joni Eareckson Tada and Steve Miller. During this time formative ideas began to take shape, which eventually would become ministries, then primary programs of *Joni and Friends*, such as *Wheels for the World*.

A genesis event in launching *Joni and Friends* as a worldwide organization occurred in Romania in 1982, for it was here and at this time that Joni refers to a clarion call of *Joni and Friends* to world missions. After viewing the desperate conditions of the impoverished Romanian people, and the even more impoverished Romanian people affected by disabilities, Joni wrote, "After a while, we looked at each other knowingly. We knew we'd seen something few Westerners were aware of. And we all felt the same thing: it was as if someone had laid a mantle on our shoulders, a burden of responsibility."[29] She added, "Years later, we would see a shocking television report on ABC's *20/20* that revealed just where all those disabled Romanian people had been during our first visit to Romania. The sunken faces of naked children–some deaf, others blind or mentally disabled–stared at the camera from filthy cribs and cold cages. . . . The images so stunned us that *Joni and Friends* launched an effort called *Wheels for the World*. It would return us to Romania with wheelchairs, physical therapists, and even more open eyes, ears, minds, and hearts."[30]

The Ministry Building Years (1990-1998)

While Joni and *Joni and Friends* were put on the world stage of missions at the 1989 Lausanne Conference in Manila, it was the first-ever International Congress on the Church and Disabilities (1990), held at Calvin College in Grand Rapids, Michigan, that officially launched the ministry into a cross-cultural world mission ministry. The impetus for Joni to be at the Manila Lausanne Conference and the 1990 Calvin College-hosted conference was that the two books, *Joni* and *A Step Further*, had been widely published in various languages around the world.

The International Congress in Grand Rapids, followed closely by the 1991 Lausanne Committee for World Evangelization in Budapest, Hungary, gave impetus to the first European Symposium on the Church and Disability, held in the Netherlands (1992). A paradigm shift occurred at this time in which the challenge was no longer solely ministry to those with disabilities by *Joni and Friends* or by challenging the church to do so. Rather, "there was a clear challenge for people with disabilities to look outwardly, to be mission minded, to be ministers of the Gospel to others."[31]

Another significant maturation of the organization's missions philosophy occurred in 1994 at the Second European Symposium on the Church and Disability. While *Joni and Friends* staff members developed, administered, and taught all of the workshops at the First European Symposium, the Second was purposely held on Eastern European soil (Budapest, Hungary), and was led and funded by Europeans with the intended purpose of "making certain it wasn't ministry, evangelism, and missions from an American perspective."[32]

The year 1993 was significant as to changes regarding U.S. operations, changes that would have implications upon missions work around the world. In 1993, *Joni and Friends* founded the first Area Ministry in Phoenix, Arizona. As Area Ministries (*Joni and Friends* outreach offices around the U.S.) began to expand in number and in ministry effectiveness, totaling eight by 2000, they also began to mobilize and train short-term mission teams from area churches to participate in *Wheels for the World* outreaches.

The official inauguration of *Wheels for the World* as a formal program began with a pioneering trip to Ghana, West Africa, in 1994. The idea of wheelchair-focused mission trips came from the 1989 Lausanne Conference in the Philippines when attendees were challenged to conduct ministry rather than only hold discussions and develop and adopt position papers. It was at this Manila conference that Joni assisted the draft of the Luke 14 disability component of the Lausanne Covenant. As a result, *Joni and Friends* shipped 150 wheelchairs for distribution, at which time the Gospel was presented to the Philippine people in their native language. Similarly, in 1991 in Moscow, Russia, during the Billy Graham Crusade, wheelchairs were again distributed, this time with Bibles.

In 1992, ten years after her first trip to Romania and in response to the
20/20 program depicting the horrible Romanian conditions for the disabled, Joni led a team back to Romania, this time with wheelchairs. It
was this trip, Joni noted, that "ratcheted up our picture of missions."
John Wern, Director of *Wheels for the World*, confirmed that "the Romanian outreach was seminal," adding that "the ministry of *Joni and
Friends* changed permanently from this time on."[33]

The 1994 *Wheels for the World* outreach to Ghana utilized wheelchairs as a means to present the Gospel while ministering to people's
physical needs through the "gift of mobility." Wern explained, "In a
previous attempt in Ghana to get people to turn out for a seminar to
bring disability ministry training, that attempt resulted in three people
attending. A seminar held in conjunction with wheelchair distribution
resulted in 130 people in attendance!"[34] The concept had been born.
Wheelchairs became the magnet of ministry, soon to become an icon of
Joni and Friends. They would become the primary means to impact millions in the next ten years. Wern explained that where foreign officials previously were indifferent, if not antagonistic, to *Joni and Friends'* efforts
before wheelchairs became a tool for evangelism, now with wheelchairs
their attitudes had totally changed. He emphasized that "from day one
our concern was to share the Gospel and leave a Bible with all wheelchair recipients and their family members. We have never wavered
from that commitment."[35] Wern wrote in 2004:

> On that inaugural outreach, 23 people delivered around 200 chairs.
> Ten years later God has expanded our ministry to global propor-
> tions, allowing us to steward a movement that has personally im-
> pacted over 2,000,000 people. The statistics themselves reveal His
> amazing handiwork. In 1994:
>
> • We had four active volunteers. Today we have close to 1,000.
> • We had no major corporate sponsors. Now we have over 7.
> • We had no facility for restoring wheelchairs. Now we have 7 pris-
>   ons restoring over 5,000 used chairs annually.
> • We had one outreach. This year we will have 13![36]

Through trial and error over the next four years, John Wern and his
team self-learned some key factors in making their wheelchair missions
program more effective:

- They made certain that indigenous churches became wheelchair distribution centers.
- They learned how to modify outreaches to fit the needs and culture of the host countries.
- They provided disability ministry and physical therapy training to native people.
- They determined that forays into foreign countries were not effective. What was needed was to establish long-term partnerships and relationships with indigenous churches and parachurch ministries and their leaders. Parallel to this was a concerted effort by *Joni and Friends'* growing number of U.S.-based Area Ministries, each committing to one country for the long haul to build in-country ministry capacity with indigenous workers and ministries.
- Noting that foreign government and non-governmental officials had become disillusioned with many missionary organizations sending "hand-me-downs" and "junk," Wern emphasized what was critically important was quality–in personnel (in-country partners and U.S. short-term missionary volunteers) and equipment, i.e., wheelchairs.

Meanwhile, in 1994 the first European office of *Joni and Friends* was established, bringing disability training seminars by Europeans to Europeans. This first European office was closed in 1999 due to financial constraints. Another lesson learned: this first foreign office looked to *Joni and Friends* in the U.S. to continue to financially support it rather than developing its own funding capacity. Irrespective of the unexpected closure of this first foreign office, the idea of foreign ministry partners representing *Joni and Friends* was an idea that would not only continue, albeit in a different format (Charters and Affiliates), but would grow in numbers.

Learning from its mistakes, instead of foreign offices under the corporate structure of *Joni and Friends* and primarily funded by *Joni and Friends*, Charters and Affiliates were started in Europe, which then spread to Africa, South America, India, and elsewhere. Charters and Affiliates are self-funded (some development assistance has been provided by *Joni and Friends* from time to time to some Charters and Affiliates), self-standing, wholly indigenous non-profit organizations established under the laws of their home countries, which are given the permission to use the "*Joni and Friends*" name in order to assist them to further their work. Lessons learned from European efforts were itemized by Joni Eareckson Tada:

- *European efforts must be led by Europeans.*
- *From the "get-go" ministries must be staffed by indigenous people.*
- *Funding must come from European sources.*
- *Donor development training is essential.*
- *Selection of leadership must come from criteria determined by nationals.*[37]

On the domestic front a search in earnest was underway in 1998 for an Executive Vice President, resulting in the hiring of Doug Mazza, now President, who filled the position in 1999. Mazza's corporate CEO and COO background with two major car manufacturing corporations, mixed with experiencing a conversion to Christ through his severely disabled son, enabled a skill set, spiritual gifting, and passion for disability ministry that provided the needed executive leadership in taking *Joni and Friends* to the next level of ministry impact. His arrival would be a harbinger of strategic changes to come in the transition years of 1999-2003.

The Transition Years (1999-2003)

Amsterdam 2000, the historic conference for evangelists from around the world hosted by the Billy Graham Association, provided the next major world stage, perhaps the largest world stage to date for Joni and disability ministry, especially in light of seeing the disability community as a distinct group to be reached for Christ. Joni's brief yet powerful plenary presentation and related workshops taught by Joni and Paul Dicken, Through The Roof Director (a London-based *Joni and Friends* Charter), created an unprecedented groundswell of demand for resources regarding ministry to people affected by disabilities. *Joni and Friends* has as of yet been unable to fully respond to the ongoing international demand for resources and training. This unprecedented demand, which continues to grow, in hindsight was prophetic in a sense–a sign to let *Joni and Friends* know that a new era was dawning for *Joni and Friends* and for disability ministry in general.

"Without God it doesn't happen," emphasized John Wern.[38] Nonetheless, God uses human beings. Wern, who has had the longest history of all *Joni and Friends* directors, referred to the 1999-2000 years as the beginning of the "Doug Mazza revolution."[39] And the arrival of Doug Mazza, President of *Joni and Friends* (then Executive Vice President), and the subsequent director level team he constructed around a new strategic plan adopted by the Board of Directors in June 2001, launched the ministry into a phenomenal season of unprecedented organizational growth and ministry fruitfulness.

Doug Mazza changed the direction of the organization's departments from a national office focus on activities and programs to a focus on serving field ministries–U.S. and international–transitioning the national office to developing programs, projects, and resources that served field ministries. As Wern noted, "Doug got our focus on the 'streets and alleys' and the 'roads and country lanes' of the Luke 14:12-24 mandate to insure that 'God's house,' the church, was full of people affected by disability. Our purpose primarily became making field ministry and churches successful in fulfilling the mandate, not becoming a bigger organization, not building our own programs."[40] Programs–*Wheels for the World*, Family Retreat, Radio, Special Delivery, and Field Ministries–that before Mazza's arrival essentially ran on separate tracks with somewhat separate agendas, increasingly became integrated. Now each program collaborates in such a way that they reinforced the others. "Synergy" in ministry and "acceleration" became key operative words, and were put increasingly in action by department directors.

Results as to this "revolution" can be seen in the following figures as reported via annual reports of each of the following departments/offices (Finance, Field Ministries, Family Retreats, *Wheels for the World*, International Operations):

- Annual cash income increased from $4.9 million at the end of 1998 to $10.5 million by the end of 2003. In 2003 the ministry raised an additional $4.9 million for its capital campaign for its permanent, first ministry-owned home–the International Disability Center.
- Field ministries (U.S.) increased from 5 Area Ministries in 1998 to 30 (10 Area Ministries, 2 Satellite Offices, 7 Ministry Associates, 9 Ministry Affiliates, and 2 Chapters) in 2003 (now 55).
- Family Retreats increased from 5 to 12 (now 16).
- *Wheels for the World* outreaches increased from 5 to 10 (14 in 2005), with the number of countries increasing from 4 to 8, and the number of wheelchairs distributed annually from 1,800 to 3,973 (5,477 in 2004).
- International operations (Charters and Affiliates) increased from 3 to 15.

In a May 2004 interview Doug Mazza attributed the growth of the ministry to several fundamental factors, not the least was the determination of the Board of Directors and Joni Eareckson Tada that the ministry was more than "about the ministry of Joni Eareckson Tada"; rather, "Joni's life was a mustard seed that was to grow a movement of ministry to those affected by disabilities . . . that the ministry is not about Joni Eareckson Tada but about what *Joni and Friends* was biblically mandated to do." He added, "The personal ministry of Joni Eareckson Tada transitioned from events, to projects, to programs, to ministry movement." He listed the key factors as:

- A clear biblical mandate following the ministry modeled by Christ to the "shut in and the shut out."
- A biblical premise that "God shows up in our weakness."
- The clear vision of Joni Eareckson Tada has kept the programs focused by being "biblically centered, evangelistic at the core, with a servant attitude to minister to people affected by disability."
- Emphasizing locally-based U.S. *Joni and Friends* field ministries as integral to what we do in developing countries by engaging the local church in our foreign outreaches, that ministry "must be executable at the community level and must involve the local church," and "field ministries must be the conduit through and by which the entire ministry is executed so that people in the field take preeminence over all programs, they drive the ministry." He added, "The chromosome of *Joni and Friends'* ministry growth is developing resources and tools for the field that are locally and culturally appropriate, providing the flexibility for local application."
- Being literal with the Luke 14 mandate to make sure the focus of ministry is to "go out to the streets and alleys . . . that we think locally and act globally."
- Staff professionalism, with all matters submitted continually to God in prayer.[41]

In summary, he emphasized that the key to *Joni and Friends'* uniqueness in quality and success is directly attributable to Joni's character, qualities, and dependence upon God. Three factors stand out:

1. "She relies and leans more on Christ than you or me due to her physical state."

2. "Though she is fallible, the practice of relying and leaning on Christ has resulted in becoming a person who makes more right decisions on a relative basis than anyone I know."
3. "She reached a Paul-like elevation of being joyful in all things . . . she is always in Paul's prison singing praises."[42]

Arguably the most crucial operating principle in creating an environment for the fruitfulness of the "Transition Years" era is revealed in one of Mazza's closing remarks during the May 16, 2004, interview: *"The most important thing leadership can provide is freedom to try and permission to fail in order to get better at what we do."*[43]

The Capstone Years (2003-5)

The second half of 2003 and 2004 have been capstone years for *Joni and Friends* as it celebrated its 25th anniversary, took note of the 10th anniversary of its premier missions program, *Wheels for the World*, and laid a foundation for accelerated international outreach in the coming decades by starting construction on its first permanent home, the *Joni and Friends* International Disability Center (IDC). By June 1 of 2005 some $8 million of the $9.3 million capital campaign goal for the Center had been raised. The IDC will not only provide the ministry much-needed office space, matching unprecedented program, project, and staffing growth, it will also house the Christian Institute on Disability inclusive of an educational adjunct, a public policy center, and a world-class training center for missionaries, churches, community organizations, and volunteers.

As statistics in the section "The Transition Years" revealed, by the end of 2003 the ministry had in less than five years more than doubled in ministry output, fruitfulness, and income. That trend continues to accelerate into 2005. For example, U.S. Field Ministries are projected to grow in number by 200% from 2006-2010.

While Joni Eareckson Tada and Doug Mazza have been providing international leadership, sharing the responsibilities as the organization's international director, a search was begun in 2004 for a qualified candidate to serve as Director of International Operations. This position is envisioned to bring together all the elements of international relations and missions under one office in order to launch an ever more aggressive, coordinated, and synergistic international outreach initiative.

It was also in 2004 that the ministry celebrated the first 10th anniversary of one of its U.S. field operations, the Phoenix Area Ministry, notable because Area Ministries are the flagship U.S.-based field ministries of *Joni and Friends*. They work locally, but reach out globally by mobilizing, equipping, training, and sending *Wheels for the World* short-term mission teams, whose members are made up of congregants from local churches.

The Years to Come (2006-)

The completion of the International Disability Center in 2006 will be much more than symbolic as to the future growth and effectiveness of the ministry. Concerning the Center, Doug Mazza noted:

- "It is an economically good decision to no longer be paying rent."
- "It puts the ministry's stake in the ground."
- "A quality home for people affected by disability speaks to the eternal home and the dignity that should be afforded the disabled in Christ."
- "It is a key element of the transition plan moving from Joni to what *Joni and Friends* does."
- "It will provide the environment for the evolution of the next part of the dream."[44]

The hiring of the first International Director of Field Operations in 2005 will complement the launch of the ministry into the next phase of Joni and Friends, which Mazza called the "era of missions and worldwide ministry." Mazza added, "It seems to me everything we have done in the last 25 years is leading us into the era of missionary work, both nationally and internationally."

CONCLUSION

In summary, it seems the growth and success of *Joni and Friends* as a missionary ministry is attributable to eight primary factors:

1. Clear calling from God.
2. A biblical mandate.
3. Christ centered.
4. Divine grace.
5. Prayer.
6. Quality character and professionalism in its leadership.

7. A focus on field ministry, not organizational growth.
8. A culture that permits and even encourages the *"freedom to try and permission to fail in order to get better at what we do."*

In her closing comments during an interview Joni Eareckson Tada summarized the ministry of *Joni and Friends* regarding the Great Commission:

> *The core of what we do is a biblical mandate. The Luke 14 mandate must be seen in the context of the Great Commission. The Gospel is for people who have lost everything. The Gospel is for the undeserving. The least and the last need to be reached. Grace is a divine initiative completely apart from man.*[45]

NOTES

1. An individual with a disability is defined as "a person who: (1) has a physical or mental impairment that substantially limits one or more major life activities, (2) has a record of such impairment, or (3) is regarded as having such impairment." (See the U.S. Equal Employment Opportunity Commission. *Facts About the Americans with Disabilities Act. http://www.eeoc.gov/facts/fs-ada.html*)

2. *The Mission of the Evangelist*, Amsterdam 2000, A Conference of Preaching Evangelists, "Reaching the Disabled," by Joni Eareckson Tada, pp. 399-400, World Wide Publications, 2000.

3. All scriptures taken from the *NIV Encouragement Bible, New International Version*, Grand Rapids, MI (Zondervan, 2001).

4. World Health Organization. *Declining Resources for Rehabilitation: A Matter of Concern.* January 30, 1996. *http://www.who.int/en/*

5. *Building Wheelchairs, Creating Opportunities*, Technology and Disability, International Perspectives, Spring 1993, Volume Two Number Two, by Henry Hof, MPA, Ralf Hotchkiss, ScD, Peter Pfaelzer, PhD. *Http://whirlwind.sfsu.edu/general_info/news_articles/building_wheelchairs/*

6. "Majority countries" refers essentially to the poor countries where the majority of the world's population lives.

7. Disability Statistics Center. *Frequently Asked Questions: How Many Americans Have A Disability? http://dsc.ucsf.edu/UCSF/spl.taf?_from=default*

8. The National Organization on Disability. *Religious Participation: Facts and Statistics. http://www.nod.org/religioun/index.cfm*

9. *Joni and Friends* grant proposal, *Opening of Closed Doors Through Disabilities Ministry*, to the Servants Charitable Trust, Dec. 6, 2001.

10. A Doctoral Thesis, by Dr. Michael Beates, Reformed Theological Seminary, March 20, 2003.

11. Lausanne Committee on World Evangelization, Manila Congress, 1989, Social Concern and Evangelism II, position papers, p. 291, *What Does the Gospel Have to Say to Disabled Persons*, by Joni Eareckson Tada.

12. Personal interview with Doug Mazza, April 15, 2004.

13. *Joni and Friends Newsletter,* 25th Anniversary, Volume 25, Number 1, January 2004.

14. As told by Judy Butler, Executive Assistant to Joni Eareckson Tada, April 30, 2004, according to her conversation with Barry Werner, formerly of World Wide Pictures.

15. *Wheels for the World* "Outreach and Distribution Numbers," April 1, 2004, a report by Samuel Buxton, Manager, *Wheels for the World.*

16. *Joni and Friends Newsletter,* "Looking Back, Pressing Forward: The Enlarged Territory of *Wheels for the World,*" Volume 25, Number 3, March 2004, p. 2.

17. Ibid.

18. *Joni and Friends Newsletter,* "Fulfilling the Great Commission: International Outreach, Short-Term Missions Partnership, and Harvest Project," Volume 25, Number 3, March 2004.

19. Personal observation of three years as Director of U.S. Field Operations of *Joni and Friends.*

20. Personal interview with Joni Eareckson Tada, March 8, 2004.

21. *Glorious Intruder, God's Presence in Life's Chaos,* by Joni Eareckson Tada, Multnomah Press, Portland, OR, 1989.

22. Faith Talk, "A Touch of Sliver–Joni Eareckson Tada Reflects on 25 Years of Ministry," Spring 2004, by Janet Chismar.

23. Personal interview with Joni Eareckson Tada, March 8, 2004.

24. *What Wondrous Love Is This,* Joni Eareckson Tada, Crossway Books, Wheaton, Ill, 2002, p. 69.

25. *The God I Love,* Joni Eareckson Tada, Zondervan, Grand Rapids, MI, 2003, p. 156.

26. *When God Weeps: Why Our Sufferings Matter to the Almighty,* by Joni Eareckson Tada and Steven Estes, Zondervan Publishing House, Grand Rapids, MI, 1997, p. 12.

27. Ibid.

28. *The God I Love,* Joni Eareckson Tada, Zondervan, Grand Rapids, MI, 2003, p. 272.

29. Ibid, p. 264.

30. Ibid, p.266.

31. Personal interview with Joni Eareckson Tada, March 8, 2004.

32. Personal interview with Joni Eareckson Tada, March 8, 2004.

33. Personal interview with John Wern, March 25, 2004.

34. Ibid.

35. Ibid.

36. *Joni and Friends Newsletter,* "Looking Back, Pressing Forward: The Enlarged Territory of Wheels for the World," Volume 25, Number 3, March 2004, p. 2.

37. Personal interview with Joni Eareckson Tada, March 8, 2004.

38. Personal interview with John Wern, March 25, 2004.

39. Ibid.

40. Ibid

41. Personal interview with Doug Mazza, April 16, 2004.

42. Ibid.

43. Ibid.

44. Ibid.

45. Personal interview, Joni Eareckson Tada, March 18, 2004.

BIBLIOGRAPHY

Beates, Michael. "Wholeness from Brokenness: Disability As A Model of the Trans-forming Power of the Gospel." Unpublished. *A Dissertation Presented to the Fac-ulty of Reformed Theological Seminary*, Orlando (2003): 11.

Buxton, Samuel. "Outreach and Distribution Numbers," a report to Joni and Friends, April 1, 2004.

Chismar, Janet. "A Touch of Sliver–Joni Eareckson Tada Reflects on 25 Years of Min-istry Faith Talk." *Faith Talk* (Spring 2004): 14-18.

Disability Statistics Center. "Frequently Asked Questions: How Many Americans Have A Disability," http://dsc.ucsf.edu/UCSF/spl.taf?_from=default

Hof, Henry, Ralf Hotchkiss, and Peter Pfaelzer. "Building Wheelchairs, Creating Op-portunities." *Technology and Disability* (Spring 1993), http://whirlwind.Sfsu.Edu/general_info/news_articles/building_wheelchairs/

Mazza, Doug. Personal interview (April 15, 2004).

Mazza, Lorraine. "Opening of Closed Doors Through Disabilities Ministry," a grant proposal to the Servants Charitable Trust, *Joni and Friends* (Dec. 6, 2001).

Tada, Joni Eareckson, and Steve Estes. *A Step Further*. Grand Rapids, MI: Zondervan, 2001.

Tada, Joni Eareckson. *Glorious Intruder, God's Presence in Life's Chaos*. Portland, Oregon: Multnomah Press, 1989.

Tada, Joni Eareckson. *Joni*. Grand Rapids, MI: Zondervan, 2001.

Tada, Joni Eareckson. Personal interview (March 8, 2004).

Tada, Joni Eareckson. "Reaching the Disabled." In *The Mission of the Evangelist, Am-sterdam 2000, A Conference of Preaching Evangelists*. Minneapolis: World Wide Publications, 2000, 399-400.

Tada, Joni Eareckson. *The God I Love*. Grand Rapids, MI: Zondervan, 2003.

Tada, Joni Eareckson. "What Does the Gospel Have to Say to Disabled Persons?" In *Lausanne Committee on World Evangelization, Manila Congress, Social Concern and Evangelism II*, position papers, Lausanne Committee, 1989, p. 291.

Tada, Joni Eareckson. *What Wondrous Love Is This*. Wheaton, IL: Crossway Books, 2002.

Tada, Joni Eareckson, and Steven Estes. *When God Weeps: Why Our Sufferings Matter to the Almighty*. Grand Rapids, MI: Zondervan, 1997.

Wern, John. "Looking Back, Pressing Forward: The Enlarged Territory of *Wheels for the World*." *Joni and Friends Newsletter* (March 2004): 2.

Wern, John. Personal interview (March 25, 2004).

World Health Organization. "Declining Resources for Rehabilitation: A Matter of Concern." http://www.who.int/en/ (January 30, 1996).

Yuen, Mike. "Fulfilling the Great Commission: International Outreach, Short-Term Missions Partnership, and Harvest Project." *Joni and Friends Newsletter* (March 2004): 5.

Yuen, Mike. "JAF Ministries, Highlights from 20 years of ministry." *Joni and Friends Newsletter* (May 1999): 4-5.

Yuen, Mike. "Radio's Reach: Transmitting Joy 'Loud and Clear!'" *Joni and Friends Newsletter* (January 2004): 7.

Mennonite Advocacy
for Persons with Disabilities

Paul D. Leichty, MDiv, BA

SUMMARY. The Mennonites, who emerged as a distinctive group from the radical wing of 16th Century Reformation, have emphasized four themes in their response to persons with disabilities: love, service, peace and justice, and community. Early ministry with children and adults with disabilities occurred within the context of family and close-knit rural community life. Work after World War II developed based on the service of Mennonite conscientious objectors in institutions for the mentally ill and developmentally disabled. Programs from then to the present developed an array of services including providing resources to congregations, operating group homes and residential facilities, and providing support to regional and church-wide arms of the church. Recent developments have focused on reorganization after changes in organizational structure and reduced funding. *[Article copies available for a fee from The Haworth Document Delivery Service: 1-800-HAWORTH. E-mail address: <docdelivery@haworthpress.com> Website: <http://www.HaworthPress.com> © 2006 by The Haworth Press, Inc. All rights reserved.]*

KEYWORDS. Mennonite, Anabaptist, group homes, reorganization

Paul D. Leichty is Director of the Anabaptist Disabilities Network (ADNet) based in Goshen, IN, and the parent of a child with developmental disabilities. A musician and ordained minister in the Mennonite Church, he has worked as an urban minister, church musician, caregiver, and advocate for persons with disabilities.

[Haworth co-indexing entry note]: "Mennonite Advocacy for Persons with Disabilities." Leichty, Paul D. Co-published simultaneously in *Journal of Religion, Disability & Health* (The Haworth Pastoral Press, an imprint of The Haworth Press, Inc.) Vol. 10, No. 1/2, 2006, pp. 195-205; and: *Disability Advocacy Among Religious Organizations: Histories and Reflections* (ed: Albert A. Herzog, Jr.) The Haworth Pastoral Press, an imprint of The Haworth Press, Inc., 2006, pp. 195-205. Single or multiple copies of this article are available for a fee from The Haworth Document Delivery Service [1-800-HAWORTH, 9:00 a.m. - 5:00 p.m. (EST). E-mail address: docdelivery@haworthpress.com].

doi:10.1300/J095v10n01_13

From the early days when Mennonites emerged as a distinctive group from the radical wing of the 16th Century Reformation known as Anabaptism, four interlocking themes formed the core of the Mennonite response to persons with disabilities.

1. An unconditional and redemptive *love* for people with special needs, based on the Biblical mandate to love all people, especially the poor, the sick, and the hurting.
2. A mandate to *serve*, acting in the name of Christ to minister healing and hope to those in need, first within the community of faith and then to the larger world.
3. A commitment to be agents of God's *peace and justice* to the earth, bringing healing to individuals, families, and nations and treating all persons with dignity and respect.
4. A sense of *community*, in which young and old, rich and poor, and those with more and less abilities could live together, experiencing God's love in an environment of safety and mutual regard, each for who he or she is.

As Mennonites increasingly engaged in the mainstream of American life starting in the late 19th and on through the 20th century, these four themes formed the basis for a Mennonite response to the needs of persons with disabilities and their families. Following World War II, Mennonites began specific ministries and organizations to express their faith in relationship to persons with disabilities, first in their own circles and then in the larger communities in which they lived.

Mennonites and Amish Mennonites (most of the latter joining or merging with Mennonite conferences in the late 19th century, leaving only the "Old Order" Amish that we know today) started migrating to North America in 1683. From then on, through most of the first half of the 20th century, the themes of love and community prevailed.

The few references that exist about the presence of persons with disabilities in the midst of mostly German-speaking Mennonite communities indicates that such persons were accepted as a part of the fabric of rural community life and put to work on the family farm doing whatever they were able to do. If there were special needs in the family due to the presence of a person with disabilities, those needs would have been handled as a matter of course by the mutual aid system administered by the deacon of the congregation.

During this time, Mennonites were largely unaware of any movements around them to care for persons with disabilities or mental illness in large institutions such as asylums and hospitals. It was natural for Mennonites who saw themselves as separate from the English-speaking world to simply care for their own people and not worry about those outside their communities. That all changed with the coming of World War II.

After experiencing considerable tensions and even persecution as a result of refusing to fight in World War I, Mennonites had joined with Brethren and Friends (Quakers) to petition the U.S. government to recognize their young men as conscientious objectors to war and allow them to perform vital services to the country that were not tied to the military. The Civilian Public Service (CPS) units established with the coming of World War II became a major test of that policy.[1] Young men were sent into some of the most wretched conditions of the deteriorating institutions for persons with mental illness and disabilities. In some cases, they were joined by their wives and other Mennonite young women. For most of these Mennonite young people coming from relatively sheltered rural environments, the experience was an immediate eye-opener. Certainly, their commitment to be agents of peace by not going to war met up with the test of whether they could perform loving service to even the most "unlovely" members of society.

While the theme of service formed the initial rationale for their actions, the experience also helped to couple the issues of justice and human dignity to the cause of peace as they joined their fellow servants in those institutions to expose the deplorable conditions that prevailed. The national exposés based on the records of these conscientious objectors were a key factor in unleashing reform movements in both the mental health and disabilities fields that followed in the last half of the twentieth century.[2]

Following the war, Mennonite mission and service institutions became involved in mental health ministries. By the early 1960s a number of community-based mental health centers opened under Mennonite sponsorship across the U.S. The work was loosely coordinated at the national level by the establishment of a Mennonite Mental Health Services (MMHS) under Mennonite Central Committee (MCC), an inter-Mennonite relief and service structure started initially in 1920 to channel relief efforts to fellow Mennonites in Russia and Ukraine.

In the midst of this work in the area of mental health, a new awareness of the needs of persons with developmental disabilities also emerged through a slightly different route. As Mennonite families increasingly moved away from the farm and into professional roles in towns and cities, the presence of a family member with disabilities took on a new dynamic within the family system. Coupled with this shift was the fact that, with advances in medicine, children with disabilities were living longer. Parents and other family members of persons with developmental disabilities began asking the larger church for help in dealing with issues such as family life activities, respite, and financial planning for adults with disabilities who outlived their parents. These families were supported by a growing number of professionals who were entering the field, largely as a result of their CPS experiences in large institutions during and after World War II.

In 1963, the concerted efforts of these families and friends in lobbying church agencies on this issue resulted in the formation by MMHS of a "Retardation Study Committee" which first met in March 1964.[3] That committee soon turned into a "Planning Committee" for a special one-day workshop held in Kansas in November 1964 in conjunction with other MMHS meetings. The focus of their concerns at this point was solely on persons that we now refer to as having "developmental disabilities" and their families.

In 1965, the Planning Committee embarked on its first project, originally envisioned by another group of parents, a special camping program at a Mennonite camp to serve persons with developmental disabilities and their families. This program was unique in that it involved the whole family. There were activities planned for both children and adults with developmental disabilities as well as any accompanying siblings. This provided not only a time of respite for parents, but also the opportunity for mutual encouragement, inspiration, and education in true community spirit. At the same time, families participated together in the retreat experience in a way that allowed "campers" to interact with each other and volunteer staff, and encouraged parents and other family members to not only learn from and support each other, but also see their children function in a different setting. This retreat has been in continuous existence at Laurelville Mennonite Church Center in Pennsylvania and is now called the "Retreat for Families, Friends, and Persons with Disabilities." Throughout the years, additional retreats using variations of this model have also taken place in other parts of the country.

The success of the camping program led to the formation of a "Resource Committee on Mental Retardation" under MMHS. The committee considered other means of educating the church and planning for additional resources and programming. Eventually, the committee became known as the "Developmental Disabilities Council." By the mid-1970s, workshops and "helps for the church" were being created under the direction of the staff of MMHS. There was also a staff consultant available to assist churches, families with a disabled member, and Mennonite-related organizations serving those with developmental disabilities.

Those organizations grew out of the same ferment as the national advocacy movement. From the start of the committee's work, the emphasis on service led to the consideration of more local community programs to serve persons with developmental disabilities. However, it was generally left to increasingly active local groups of parents in strong Mennonite communities to create the organizations that would care for their loved ones after they were gone. Their concern was primarily that their loved ones would have a wholesome Christian community with proper supports after they, as an increasingly mobile extended family system, were no longer able to care for them. Today, disability services providers with ties to Mennonite churches exist in Pennsylvania, Maryland, Virginia, Ohio, Indiana, Missouri, Oregon, and California with an additional project emerging in Arizona.

Most of these organizations focus on residential services for adults with developmental disabilities. The main model used is that of the group home where four to eight persons live together in a household along with caregivers. In many places, live-in caregivers have been the norm as married couples or groups of two or three single persons live with the residents. This model has worked best when residents functioned well enough to do all their own personal care and had work or day programs to which they could go during working hours. This allowed a caregiving couple, for example, to take at least one outside job between them during those same hours and thus support themselves. For the organizations, this reduced costs.

Typically, such caregivers saw their work as fitting in with the post-war pattern of "Voluntary Service" (VS). VS emerged as one alternative service option for young men of draft age during the period of military conscription that lasted through the Vietnam War era. Young adults in general were encouraged to give a period of up to two years to VS and even young married couples just out of college were involved. For some, VS became a more long-term lifestyle, and caregiving in Mennonite-sponsored group homes became an avenue of service. Even older couples in a life transition or newly retired seniors have participated in this movement.

However, as the draft ended and more young adults went right into college and then into the kind of jobs that enabled them to pay off their college loans, more and more caregivers came from outside of the church. In many cases, the service providers needed to pay a more standard wage, provide the time off needed to avoid burnout, or go to a modified or full shift rotation to staff the homes. This led to more service providers turning to government funding to provide ongoing residential services.

Some Mennonite-related service providers also have vocational and day activity programs and have been part of a movement to encourage companies to employ persons with disabilities. Typically, these programs also rely on government funding. However, for all of the service provider programs, there are also fundraising efforts within the local communities to make up the difference between what the government provides and what is necessary to sustain a wholesome quality of community life for the persons being served.

In 1978 the role of the Developmental Disabilities Council changed from that of advisor to MMHS to an "administrative" and "policy setting" role. This allowed for the hiring in 1979 of the first full-time staff devoted exclusively to disabilities resources. By this time, MCC, as the parent organization, was more focused on peace and justice issues and this emphasis carried over into the advocacy work for disabilities. Questions were raised as to whether the developmental disabilities work should broaden to include the needs of families and individuals with other types of disabilities, including mental illness.

With designated staff and administrative and a policy-setting board, the advocacy ministries in the '80s were known as Mennonite Developmental Disability Services (MDDS). As MCC itself decentralized its operations and opened regional offices, developmental disabilities committees sprang up in each MCC region. These committees were instrumental in linking the concerns of families in the congregations to the advocacy ministries. Some of these regional committees were active in establishing new service provider organizations in their regions. It is worth noting that in one case, MCC West Coast, a full-time staff position was designated to serve in disabilities ministry. At the national level MDDS provided a coordinating role for these regional committees and also served as a forum for locally controlled service providers around the country to build networks of support and encouragement.

During this time, a parallel national advocacy program developed around the issues of mental illness. By this time, the mental health service providers themselves had become strong multi-service community agencies, locally operated and funded largely by fees and government funding. However, there was not generally a strong connection to Mennonite churches and therefore, there had not been much attention paid to education and advocacy around the issues of mental illness at the congregational level. MDDS provided a model for that to happen for mental illness as well through the Mental Health Awareness and Education Program (MHA&EP).

During the 1970s and '80s, MDDS worked diligently to provide resources for families and congregations. A Disabilities Awareness Sunday was added to the church calendar and resource packets of worship and educational materials were created annually. With the assistance of lawyers within the church, guidelines and principles were developed to aid parents in planning for their loved ones after their death. Increasingly, the theme of community came to the forefront as congregations were given models and encouraged to form circles of care for each adult with a disability in order to provide the ongoing community of support that would leave parents feeling at peace about the future. The little booklet entitled "Supportive Care in the Congregation" is still in print. Even though few congregations have implemented all of the details in the plan, it has nevertheless served as a model and inspiration for thinking about these issues from the standpoint of the wider family of faith instead of just the biological family.

With the coming of the last quarter of the 20th century, MCC and the various Mennonite regional and national mission agencies gradually realized that they were administering many scattered health and human service organizations on parallel tracks. Included among these organizations were a growing number of nursing homes and retirement communities, as well as providers of disabilities services. Mission boards particularly wanted to turn over the administration of local service provider organizations to the local community. At the same time, there was a keen desire on the part of many that these local organizations to retain a distinctive Mennonite witness through some kind of linkage with the church structures. In 1988, MMHS was renamed "Mennonite Health Services" (MHS) and given the mandate to guide and serve these local community health and human service providers of all types. This was further encouragement for locally-controlled disability services providers to see their services as related to the national and binational church.

As MHS grew to become a distinctive entity from MCC, its role became increasingly more focused as a resource to the self-supporting local agencies which it served. This led to the question about the relationship of MHS to the disabilities and mental health advocacy ministries. The advocacy ministries were not bound to a local geographic area, serving families and congregations directly throughout the country. They also relied, for the most part, on donated funds. In the early '90s, as a formal separation was planned between MCC and MHS, the question of the placement of the advocacy programs within either of the parent organizations remained in limbo.

The disabilities and mental illness advocacy programs fell victim to a complex set of forces. Mission boards were clear that their mission was not in administering intricate health care structures and were increasingly focusing on planting new churches and resourcing churches for spiritual outreach both overseas and at home. MCC, with its emphasis on cutting-edge peace and justice ministries that had originally strengthened the advocacy programs, now moved on to other issues. The divestiture of MHS made the MCC governing board reluctant to welcome the disabilities and mental illness advocacy ministries which they assumed were a remnant of the old health care organization administration system. At the same time, MHS felt a need and mandate to serve the local service organizations, relying on their membership dues for funding. The church-wide advocacy ministries, with no steady funding source or administrative structure to benefit from MHS resources simply did not fit into this new scheme.

In 1994, with MHS established apart from MCC, a decision had to be made regarding a "home" for the advocacy ministries. Mennonite Mutual Aid (MMA), a stewardship ministry of the Mennonite Church (and other Anabaptist-related denominations) stepped forward and agreed to sponsor the programs. Accepting these ministries was a "stretch" for MMA as their mission was focused on developing stewardship education and wellness education resources and products. MCC eased the transition by promising a level of funding that would decrease over five years.

Historically, MMA has held the Mennonite Church mandate to provide affordable health insurance to church members. However, as they increasingly faced financial pressures in a complex and constantly changing national health care environment in the '70s and '80s, MMA's energies went increasingly into providing general stewardship products and health awareness and education efforts at the congregational level through a system of congregational advocates. This was coupled with a stewardship emphasis related to its investment products (mutual funds, foundation investments, etc.). The result was that the advocacy programs for disabilities and mental illness were seen as two expansions in MMA's "Stewardship Education" emphasis.

The initial result was a flurry of activity around the development of tangible disability and mental illness "products" that could be marketed to families and congregations to help offset the costs of this ministry. At the same time, the tradition of mutual aid and donor support made MMA reluctant to move whole-heartedly into a marketing approach. Updated and new materials were produced and the two half-time consultants, hired by MMA to replace the earlier advocacy staff, spent considerable energy getting into conference and congregational settings. In addition, extra efforts were made to connect again with families as a consultant was hired to revive the flagging disabilities retreat at Laurelville and develop new retreats for family members of persons with mental illness.

At the same time, the national committees that had earlier set policy were downgraded to advisory status and then eliminated altogether in a cost-cutting move. MCC regional committees on developmental disabilities gradually faded as well since they were no longer tied back to the parent organization. MMA's volunteer, congregationally-based advocacy system was able to pick up some of the slack of congregational connectedness, but the effect was more diffuse without committees of activists meeting regularly.

Even given these significant changes, the mental illness and disability advocacy programs did adapt to MMA's environment and ran smoothly during the stock market boom of the late 1990s and early into the new millennium. As MCC's subsidies ended in 1999, a meeting was called in early 2000 for MMA, MCC US, and MHS to evaluate the future of the programs. MCC US continued to encourage its regional organizations to have disabilities programs of their choosing, but did not pursue creating anything on the national level, despite the fact that MCC Canada continued to sponsor the disabilities and mental health advocacy programs in that country. MHS reaffirmed its position that the programs did not belong in its organizational structure and MMA agreed to continue to sponsor them without the MCC subsidies.

The clash of the stewardship theme with the earlier themes of love, service, peace and justice, and community finally took its toll. As the stock market turned sour and health care costs continued to put pressure on its revenue-producing insurance programs, MMA decided it needed to focus on its stewardship core. MMA made a unilateral decision and the advocacy programs were eliminated on short notice at the end of September 2002.

Yet, a small group of parents in Indiana, site of MMA's offices, picked up the banner. After making contacts with MHS, service providers, and officials from Mennonite Church USA, the ad hoc committee determined that there was no church agency willing to pick up sponsorship of the advocacy programs even though they all agreed there was a need for them. So this group of parents called together a larger group of parents, individuals with disabilities, and friends and were empowered to form a new organization to carry on the work.

The Anabaptist Disabilities Network (ADNet) was thus formed in early 2003. MMA agreed to give the fledgling group its remaining stock of disability and mental illness resource materials and provide some initial funding for start-up costs. A national Board was recruited and met for the first time in January 2004. By mid-summer of that year, volunteer efforts were waning and fundraising was going well enough to hire a half-time Director starting in September. MMA continued to be supportive by providing a matching grant to donated funds.

ADNet has continued to distribute resource materials published by MMA, some of which date back to the MCC days. It has continued to publish a periodic newsletter directed to this constituency and initiated new communications through a Web site, a toll-free voice mail system, and a quarterly electronic newsletter for congregations. Presentations have been given in a number of area churches in worship and Sunday school settings.

In 2004, ADNet responded to nearly 90 requests for information and resourcing from individuals, families, congregations, and church-related agencies in 22 states. These requests included booklets on topics ranging from estate planning and "Supportive Care in the Congregation" to essays on "A Christian View of Mental Illness." Also provided were videos from a loan library, accessibility audits, and referrals to Mennonite service provider organizations. ADNet also participates (as did its immediate predecessor) in the loosely structured National Council of Churches of Christ Committee on Disabilities. This connection, along with the increased exposure of the Website, have resulted in other denominations outside of the Anabaptist community also using ADNet's materials.

Future goals for ADNet include better utilization of electronic discussion groups as well as linkages with and the establishment of more local and regional face-to-face support groups. ADNet would also like to build a centralized database by which individuals, families, and congregations could gain ready access to people, media, and organizational resources in the style of a true network. This would include a national network of consultants to congregations on accessibility issues.

ADNet has emphasized the effort of congregations to build community that includes all persons regardless of their abilities. However, just as at the beginning of the advocacy efforts for persons with disabilities, the ministry is again being championed by families and individuals living with disabilities and mental illness. This group continues to remind the church that the themes that the church holds dear, peace, justice, and community, apply to persons with disabilities and need to be fleshed out in concrete actions of love and service.

NOTES

1. This story is told through a PBS film entitled "The Good War and Those Who Refused to Fight It" and accompanying website at *http://www.pbs.org/itvs/thegoodwar/*

2. Sareyan, Alex. The Turning Point: How Persons of Conscience Brought About Major Change in the Care of America's Mentally Ill. Pennsylvania: Herald Press, 1994.

3. From here on, source materials for this article consist mainly of archival papers housed in the offices of ADNet and in the Mennonite Church USA archives, both located in Goshen, IN.

Working Interfaith: The History of the Religion and Disability Program of the National Organization on Disability

Albert A. Herzog, Jr., PhD, MDiv, MA

SUMMARY. This article traces the history of the Religion and Disability Program of the National Organization on Disability from its inception in 1989 to the present. Over the years, its goal has been to identify and remove barriers to the full participation of worshipers with disability. Program activities include the publication of guides such as *That All May Worship*, *Loving Justice*, and *From Barriers to Bridges*, the cosponsoring of over 225 "That All May Worship" conferences across America, the Accessible Congregation Campaign and the Seminary Project. In all these and more, the program has sought to promote full inclusion of persons with disabilities by emphasizing the gifts and talents of children and adults with disabilities and the need for all religious communities (congregations, denominations, faith groups, and seminaries) to be accessible and welcoming. *[Article copies available for a fee from The Haworth Document Delivery Service: 1-800-HAWORTH. E-mail address: <docdelivery@ haworthpress.com> Website: <http://www.HaworthPress.com> © 2006 by The Haworth Press, Inc. All rights reserved.]*

Albert A. Herzog, Jr. is a Lecturer in Sociology at the Ohio State University, Newark, as well as an ordained minister in the United Methodist Church.

[Haworth co-indexing entry note]: "Working Interfaith: The History of the Religion and Disability Program of the National Organization on Disability." Herzog, Albert A. Jr. Co-published simultaneously in *Journal of Religion, Disability & Health* (The Haworth Pastoral Press, an imprint of The Haworth Press, Inc.) Vol. 10, No. 1/2, 2006, pp. 207-226; and: *Disability Advocacy Among Religious Organizations: Histories and Reflections* (ed: Albert A. Herzog, Jr.) The Haworth Pastoral Press, an imprint of The Haworth Press, Inc., 2006, pp. 207-226. Single or multiple copies of this article are available for a fee from The Haworth Document Delivery Service [1-800-HAWORTH, 9:00 a.m. - 5:00 p.m. (EST). E-mail address: docdelivery@haworthpress.com].

Available online at http://www.haworthpress.com/web/JRDH
© 2006 by The Haworth Press, Inc. All rights reserved.
doi:10.1300/J095v10n01_14

KEYWORDS. National Organization on Disability, N. O. D., Religion and Disability Program, interfaith action, *That All May Worship*, accessibility, welcoming, congregational accessibility, A Ramp is Not Enough

Since 1989, the Religion and Disability Program of the National Organization on Disability (N. O. D.) has advocated for accessible places of worship of all faiths and the full inclusion of people with disabilities in the congregations of their choice. "Today," as the 2001 Annual Report of N. O. D. suggests, "the program is grandly fulfilling its original mission: identifying and helping to remove barriers to the full participation of worshipers with disabilities."[1] Such a bold assessment is easy to document as the work has taken its many forms–from gaining access to congregations to including issues of disability on the agendas of theological seminaries. Its contribution to the inclusion of people with disabilities into mainstream American life is found in the events which have unfolded over the years since the program's inception.

N.O. D. emerged in the aftermath of the 1981 International Year of Disabled Persons (IYDP) declared by the United Nations. The IYDP called upon all nations to recognize their citizens with disabilities, many of whom "were doubly disadvantaged by poverty" and urged "governments, communities, religions, and organizations to adopt the IYDP goal of full and equal participation of people with disabilities in all aspects of life."[2] In response, the U. S. Council for IYDP was formed as "the first private sector group in any country to fund and lead a U. N. International Year observance." It quickly built a staff of 30 to provide oversight for the observance, and at the year's conclusion, representatives from 48 states met in Washington, D.C., and established the National Office on Disability to "continue the momentum toward the IYDP's goal. In 1983, the name was changed to the National Organization on Disability (N. O. D.)"[3]

The events of the IYDP were extended by the proclamation "America's Goals for the International Decade of Disabled Persons, 1983-1992 as stated in Resolution 39 of the United States Congress." Over the ten year period, various organizations, including N. O. D., sought to "foster public understanding, full participation and acceptance of disabled persons" through:

– Expanded Educational Opportunity.
– Improved Access to Housing, Buildings, and Transportation.

- Expanded Participation in Recreational, Social, Religious, and Cultural Activities.
- Expanded and Strengthened Rehabilitation Programs and Facilities.
- Purposeful Application of Biomedical Research Aimed at Conquering Major Disabling Conditions.
- Reduction of the Incidence of Disability by Expanded Accident and Disease Prevention.
- Increased Application of Technology to Minimize the Effects of Disability.
- Expanded International Exchange of Information and Experience to Benefit All Disabled Persons.[4]

In keeping with these goals, the Board of N. O. D. was composed of national business and civic leaders with a keen interest in integrating people with disabilities into the mainstream. One such person was the Reverend Harold Wilke who had a long career as a United Church of Christ minister and disability advocate. He knew, first-hand, that places of worship were inaccessible and largely unwelcoming to people with disabilities and raised, at a regular Board meeting, the need for an on-going effort to facilitate their inclusion into all aspects of religious life. In 1987 and 1988, N. O. D. sought to establish "a concentrated effort to promote and expand the participation of disabled persons in the religious life of their communities, emphasizing greater accessibility of places of worship and the involvement of disabled persons in the activities of their places or worship."[5]

The 1989 action by the N. O. D. Board of Directors establishing the Religion and Disability Program built upon N. O. D.'s original intent to make religious participation of people with disabilities a major priority. The decision to develop a major programmatic thrust linking religion and disability was a milestone for its effort to remove architectural and attitudinal barriers through interfaith action. With the Board approval, N. O. D. employed Ginny Thornburgh as Director of the Religion and Disability Program. Ms. Thornburgh, wife of the former Governor of Pennsylvania and former United States Attorney General, Dick Thornburgh, had first-hand experience as an advocate for her son with disability. She had worked extensively with the Association for Retarded Citizens (now The Arc), and served as the first disability coordinator for Harvard University. In addition, her experience as an educator enabled her to foster awareness of disability issues among religious leaders with a common sense approach.

One year after the Religion and Disability Program was established, two significant events occurred which illustrate the effective linkage of its program and its director. In December 1990, a press conference at N. O. D.'s Washington, D. C. office drew "important and strong media attention." Ginny Thornburgh had just returned from the Vatican and a personal audience with Pope John Paul II where she proposed "Vatican sponsorship of an International Conference in 1992 on 'Persons with Disabilities' for the purpose of meeting the church's worldwide responsibility to increase the participation of people with disabilities in congregations." She reported that the Vatican had agreed to give her proposal "serious attention."[6]

This event followed a series of contacts made prior to the establishment of the Religion and Disability Program and the hiring of Ms. Thornburgh as its director. Alan Reich, N. O. D.'s President and a wheelchair user, had visited the Vatican on June 17, 1987, where, in an audience with Pope John Paul II, he urged the issuing of a Papal Encyclical on persons with disabilities. In his presentation before the Holy Father, he noted that the Pope's first "Encyclical on Redemption" was a "beacon of hope for all humanity" as humankind entered the "Bi-millennium Era." He also noted that in the Pope's statement in Canada on September 10, 1984, special attention was called to "persons with physical or mental disabilities" and the "imperative for including disabled persons in religious and secular life and for enlarging their contribution to society."[7] He urged the Pontiff to acknowledge the need for every person with a disability to "participate in the everyday life of the community." He then urged the Pope to "usher in the new Millennium in a more human and humane way, [since] you, uniquely in the world, can renew the dream and promise of the U. N. Decade of Disabled Persons." Mr. Reich, as President of N. O. D., issued an appeal for His Holiness to:

> Continue and enunciate a Series of Bi-millennium Encyclicals through issuing at the United Nations later this year–at the mid-point of U. N. Decade of Disabled Persons–an Encyclical on mankind and disability, building on and reinforcing your encyclicals to date, by calling upon the United Nations, governments at all levels, religious, organizations, institutions, communities, and people of good will everywhere to strive toward and achieve the aims of the United Nations Decade of Disabled Persons.

He continued by listing the impact of such a statement which would:

a. Reinforce the worldwide process you have begun in a very human way of utilizing the Bi-millennium turning point at the year 2000 as a humanizing, civilizing force for love, truth, justice, and equality.
b. Help and inspire disabled people everywhere by focusing attention on the need for commitment and action in the name of the United Nations Decade of Disabled Persons, its goals, and thereby calling for full participation, as well as charity, as appropriate in the various countries of the world.
c. Strengthen confidence in the United Nations itself by projecting to the world that the U. N. is helping build, through such initiatives as the U. N. Decade of Disabled Persons, the human foundations of the structure of peace.[8]

This event set the tone for the Religion and Disability Program as it sought to integrate religious issues within the mainstream effort for the total inclusion of people with disabilities in every aspect of social life.

In addition, the Religion and Disability Program sought to do its share in fostering greater acceptance of people with disabilities among congregations of all faiths. In 1990, it received funding from the Scaife Family Foundation and the J. M. Foundation to "provide for the preparation and distribution of an interfaith handbook to assist denominational groups, seminaries and local congregations to become more welcoming to persons with disabilities."[9] Also, Ms. Thornburgh appeared as a guest on Dr. Robert Schuller's television program, *Hour of Power* and addressed numerous "lay and religious groups on the need for making places of worship more accepting of and accessible to persons with disabilities."[10]

By the end of 1992, N. O. D. had not only published its handbook *That All May Worship: An Interfaith Welcome to People with Disabilities*, but issued its second printing of 15,000 copies.[11] The handbook became known not only for what it says about accessibility, but for how it says it. Within its 52 pages are lists describing how a congregation–of any faith–can develop a program to remove architectural barriers as well as provide the hospitality necessary to make persons with various disabilities at home in places of worship. Rather than long descriptive narratives, the handbook offers short bullets of information designed to grab the reader's attention, thereby encouraging creative responses tailored to specific congregational needs. The narratives are interspersed with photographs of persons with disabilities doing things in actual congregations, and with pithy scriptural texts and other quotations all designed, again, to provoke thought and creative responses rather than an itemized list of do's and don'ts. The handbook is dedicated to the late Reverend Harold Wilke who is pictured on page iii with others at the signing into law of the Americans With Disabilities Act in 1990. He is shown reaching out with his foot (he has no arms) to receive a pen from President George H. W. Bush.[12]

In November, 1992, N. O. D. president Alan Reich, board member Reverend Harold Wilke, and Religion and Disability Program director Ginny Thornburgh traveled to Rome to address the first Vatican international conference on disability. In addition to Pope John Paul II, 80 speakers from around the world participated in the conference attended by 9,000 people. One of the sponsors of the conference was the World Committee on Disability which, since 1997, operated "as an adjunct of N. O. D. and as one of several efforts at the international level designed to enhance action with and on behalf of people with disabilities around the world as part of the United Nations Decade of Disabled Persons."[13]

The year 1993 was also another year of growth for the Religion and Disability Program. The N. O. D. Annual Report indicated that "nearly 20,000 copies of its handbook *That All May Worship* had been sold and distributed since its initial publication in June, 1992." The handbook was featured in "both *Modern Maturity*, a publication of the American Association of Retired Persons (AARP), with a circulation of more than 2.2 million readers nationwide, and in *Guideposts*, with 4 million subscribers."[14] During 1993 and 1994, N. O. D. held the first "That All May Worship" conferences in eight cities in California, Oklahoma, Connecticut, Pennsylvania, South Carolina, and Georgia. The insights gained at these conferences would serve as the basis for a new publication entitled *From Barriers to Bridges: A Community Action Guide for Congregations and People with Disabilities* released in 1994. Indeed, the Religion and Disability Program had already secured another grant from the Scaife Family Foundation to cover the publication costs of this second guide.[15]

The 1994 Annual Report of the National Organization on Disability opened its section on "Creating Welcoming Congregations" by stating that:

> N. O. D.'s Religion and Disability Program, launched more than five years ago, is now solidly established. Although there are other programs across the nation urging that people with disabilities be served by a specific faith group, N. O. D. alone is interfaith, respecting and connecting with a variety of religious traditions and

disability organizations. N. O. D.'s religion program has two guiding beliefs:

- *Places of Worship should welcome everyone*
- *People with disabilities have gifts to bring to their congregations*[16]

The report also noted that since its publication in mid-1992, "more than 25,000 copies of N. O. D's handbook, *That All May Worship*, have been distributed nationwide. In addition, the October, 1993 *Guideposts* article describing it has been reprinted in several places, including the December, 1994 issue of *Exceptional Parent* magazine."[17]

In 1994, N. O. D. published a "companion handbook" entitled *Loving Justice: The ADA and the Religious Community*. As described in the Annual Report: "This 36-page resource guide describes how portions of the Americans With Disabilities Act, including the Title I employment provisions, affect religious institutions, including congregations, hospitals, nursing homes, seminaries, universities, colleges, schools, camps, and social service agencies." Funds for printing *Loving Justice* also were made possible by a grant from the Scaife Family Foundation which had "provided major support to N. O. D.'s Religion and Disability Program since its inception." The Annual Report also noted that "the guide had been well received by leaders in the disability, religious, and legal communities."[18]

Featured in the 1994 report is a picture of the Reverend Harold Wilke seated on the floor autographing a copy of his book *Creating the Caring Congregation* during an N. O. D. "That All May Worship" conference. The autograph was done with his foot and there is a quote from Rev. Wilke in caption format: "A ramp is not enough."[19]

In 1995, the "Creating Welcoming Congregations" section of the N. O. D. Annual Report once again pointed to "That All May Worship" as the central theme of the Religion and Disability Program. Through the assistance of Dr. Young Woo Kang, a member of the N. O. D. World Committee on Disability, *That All May Worship* was translated into Korean and distributed to religious organizations throughout the Republic of Korea.[20] Also reported was information about *From Barriers to Bridges* which was "designed to foster dialogue and cooperation among people with disabilities, their family members, religious leadership, and the larger community." It was designed to provide the "detailed guidance needed to hold a 'That All May Worship' conference and other community-building activities."[21] Included in this long-awaited publication were numerous cartoons exposing the ignorant but often humorous ways that ordinary persons approach people with disabilities.

The 1996 Annual Report of N. O. D. reiterated that "many people with disabilities find places of worship not as accessible or welcoming as they could be."[22] In fact, two years earlier, N. O. D. commissioned Louis Harris and Associates, Inc. of New York to conduct a survey entitled *N. O. D./Harris Survey of Americans with Disabilities*. In that survey conducted February 3 through March 3, 1994, the Harris poll found that "half of all adults with disabilities (49%) attend church or synagogue at least once a month, and 12% attend religious services less than once a month." "These attendance levels," the Report noted, "are lower than among adults with no disabilities; a majority (58%) of adults without disabilities attend church or synagogue at least once a month."[23] In addition, the Report stated that:

> Among both adults with and without disabilities, roughly one in ten (9% and 11% respectively) is a frequent visitor, going to a place of worship at least twice a week. Adults with disabilities are more likely to never visit a church or synagogue (39%) than to make visits less than once a month (12%). Adults without disabilities are more often occasional visitors (20%) as compared to those with disabilities, and they are less likely to never go to a church or synagogue (22%). Younger adults with disabilities, as compared with their older peers, are more likely to make occasional visits to a place of worship. Nearly half (46%) of seniors 75 years old or older with disabilities never visit a church or synagogue.[24]

These data indicated and supported the on-going need for the Religion and Disability Program's emphasis on urging "local congregations, national denominational groups, and seminaries to remove architectural, communication and attitudinal barriers."[25] And in response, The Religion and Disability Program continued to emphasize its sponsorship of "That All May Worship" conferences throughout America. These were "community-building conferences [designed to] bring together people with disabilities and religious leadership to plan improved access–both physical and spiritual–in houses of worship." With eight sponsored in 1996, the grand total of conferences held was brought to 22. The *1996 N. O. D. Annual Report* indicated that "conference sites have been as diverse as churches, synagogues, community colleges, rehabilitation hospitals, senior citizens' centers and seminaries. The conferences have ranged in size from 60 to 600 and have informed and motivated a wide range of participants, with and without disabilities."[26]

The assertion that the "conferences inspire congregations to take further actions that will improve access" was confirmed by the fact that "as a direct result of the September, 1996 Birmingham, Alabama conference, one congregation held a three-week series about ministry and disability, several congregations held a 'Disability Awareness Day,' and one congregation formed a Disability Task Force. And, similar initiatives are in the works throughout the U.S. as a result of 'That All May Worship' Conferences."[27] This conviction was further enhanced by a picture to the left of the report which featured Ginny Thornburgh with the late theologian Father Henri Nouwen and the late His Eminence, Joseph Cardinal Bernardin at the Chicago "That All May Worship" Conference. Below was a picture of Ginny Thornburgh presenting a copy of the guide *That All May Worship* to members of the University Christian Church of Hyattsville, Maryland.[28]

During 1997, "That All May Worship" conferences were held in 22 communities "from Hillsboro, Oregon to Melville, New York and Mankato, Minnesota to Winfield, Alabama." Philadelphia's "That All May Worship" conference led to the establishment of an ongoing "That All May Worship Network." People from a variety of faiths "formed this network to work toward the goal of full religious access throughout the Greater Philadelphia area."[29]

The 1998 N. O. D. Annual Report noted significant milestones as the Religion and Disability Program moved toward the year 2000. Under the heading "Working with Congregations and Communities," the program reported that it "works with congregations, national denominational groups, and seminaries to remove architectural, communication and attitudinal barriers." A total of 23 "That All May Worship" conferences were held during the year in locations "from Tacoma, Washington to Fall River, Massachusetts–from Chicago, Illinois to Lakeland, Florida" all in an effort to "foster dialogue among people with disabilities, concerned citizens, and religious leaders as they work to improve physical and spiritual access in their congregation."[30] Also reported was a speaking tour to the Republic of Korea by Ginny Thornburgh and her husband Dick which was hosted by Dr. and Mrs. Young Woo Kang. Dr. Kang was then Vice Chairman, N. O. D.'s World Committee on Disability and a member of N. O. D.'s Board of Directors.[31]

However, the most significant event in 1998 for the Religion and Disability Program was the launching of the Accessible Congregations

Campaign, "the goal of which [was] to recruit 2,000 committed congregations by the year 2000 that include people with disabilities as full and active participants." The Campaign was supported by eighty-five organizations including the National Down Syndrome Society, the Jewish Educational Service of North America and the National Council on Independent Living and had as its theme "Access: It Begins in the Heart."[32] This effort was aimed directly at "congregations of all faiths and is based on the scriptural understanding that people, with and without disabilities, are created in the image of God" as "Point 3" of *Ten Things You Should Know About the Accessible Congregations Campaign*, indicated. This list was included along with a "Commitment Form" and a "Certificate" that were distributed to congregations, denominations and faith groups. The fourth through tenth items on the "Ten Things You Should Know" list indicate the depth of the Program's efforts to promote accessible congregations:

4. The campaign seeks to identify and certify the full range of congregations–from those newly alert to disability issues to those which are architecturally and programmatically accessible.
5. An Accessible Congregation acknowledges that it has barriers (both physical and attitudinal) to the full participation of people with disabilities and *makes a commitment* to removing them.
6. *Congregations need not be perfect.* They do need to set achievable goals and make a commitment to action.
7. To join the campaign, a congregation must commit to using the gifts and talents of people with disabilities in worship, service, study, and leadership. A congregation then completes and returns the Commitment Form to Lorraine Thal, Coordinator, Accessible Congregations Campaign at N. O. D., 910 Sixteenth Street, NW, Washington, DC 20006.
8. N. O. D. will then send the congregation a certificate suitable for display.
9. Joining the ACC costs nothing. The brochure, information packet, and commitment certificate are *free.*
10. The N. O. D. Web site at *www.nod.org/religion* lists committed congregations by state.[33]

The Certificate had a number of features including: a special logo; a quotation from the Old Testament Prophet Isaiah 56:7–"for my house shall be called a house of prayer for all peoples"; a place for the name of the congregation; and a place for a date and signatures for both Ginny

Thornburgh as Director of the Religion and Disability Program and Lorraine Thal as Coordinator of the Accessible Congregations Campaign.[34] The certificate contains three principles concerning the congregation which has "committed to include people with disabilities as full and active participants in this Accessible Congregation":

> In this congregation, people with disabilities are valued as individuals, having been created in the image of God.
>
> This congregation is endeavoring to remove barriers of architecture, communications, and attitude that excluded people with disabilities from full and active participation
>
> People, with and without disabilities, are encouraged in this congregation to practice their faith and use their gifts in worship, service, study, and leadership.[35]

In speeches, articles, e-mails and telephone calls, Ginny Thornburgh and Lorraine Thal talked about the right to a full life of faith for children and adults with disabilities–including worship, service, study, and leadership. At the end of 1999, 970 congregations across America had committed to the Accessible Congregations Campaign. Within the 1999 Annual Report was a statement: *"Computers Aren't The Only Things That Need Updating For The New Millennium–Our Places of Worship Do, Too."* Underneath the Campaign logo was the following invitation: "Join the Accessible Congregations Campaign and be one of the 2,000 congregations of all faiths committed to welcoming people with disabilities in the year 2000."[36]

This focus, while adding a new and significant direction to The Religion and Disability Program, did not sideline the emphasis which had been in place for ten years. Numerous "That All May Worship" conferences were held around the country and the three guides–*That All May Worship, Loving Justice,* and *From Barriers to Bridges* continued to "serve as invaluable resources to congregations of all faiths wishing to expand the participation of people with disabilities."[37]

Two additional and interesting items were contained in the 1999 Annual Report. The Religion and Disability Program received a grant from the W. H. Kellogg Foundation in support of the Accessible Congregations Campaign. Also included was a quotation from its Director, Ginny Thornburgh. At a "That All May Worship" conference in Bethlehem, Pennsylvania, she indicated that "a ramp is not enough. We must be about the business of disregarding old attitudes about people with disabilities and open ourselves to their potential."[38]

During the year 2000, "the Accessible Congregations Campaign continued its efforts to enroll congregations that make the commitment to removing barriers and to welcoming people with disabilities into a full life of faith." And, while the goal of "two-thousand congregations by 2000" would not be achieved until 2001, N. O. D's Religion and Disability Program continued to stress its distribution of resource materials as well as the holding of "That All May Worship" conferences across the United States. Its leading publication, *That All May Worship*, was now in its sixth edition with over 50,000 copies having been distributed since its first printing. Twenty-one "That All May Worship" conferences were held during the year, bringing to 116 the total number held between 1993 and 2000.[39] The title for the Religion and Disability Program section of N.O.D.'s 2000 Annual Report was "Closing the Gap: In Religious Participation."[40]

The National Organization on Disability marked the year 2001 with several "high notes" which would either directly or indirectly affect The Religion and Disability Program. After N. O. D.'s six-year campaign to add a statue of President Franklin Delano Roosevelt in his wheelchair at the FDR Memorial in Washington, D.C., the statue was dedicated by President Clinton who called it a "reminder for all who touch, who see, who wheel and walk around they, too, are free."[41] Two weeks later, N. O. D. was working with the new administration of President George W. Bush who announced the New Freedom Initiative which would in the view of N. O. D. represent "a broad-based commitment to advance the full participation of people with disabilities in American life."[42] In addition, N. O. D. worked, actively, to assure plans for emergency preparedness (in the wake of the terrorist acts of September 11th) for the disability community.[43]

The Religion and Disability Program enrolled the 2,000th congregation in N. O. D.'s Accessible Congregations Campaign early in 2001. The Adas Israel Congregation of Washington, D.C. hosted the celebration of achieving the program goal of 2,000 congregations. The congregation which held the distinguished position of the 2,000th congregation enrolled was the First United Methodist Church of Germantown (Philadelphia), Pennsylvania. The complete list of participating congregations was posted by state on the N. O. D. website at *www.nod.org/religion* and plans were laid to continue adding committed congregations to the list.[44]

Another significant milestone was achieved with the publication of the booklet, *Money and Ideas: Creative Approaches to Congregational Access*. The publication was prepared in cooperation with the Alban Institute and "describes creative initiatives and fundraising strategies used by 50 congregations to maximize accessibility." This added to the list of publications including *That All May Worship*, *Loving Justice*, and *From Barriers to Bridges*.[45]

As the Religion and Disability Program looked ahead to 2002, it laid plans to "focus on seminaries by facilitating conferences on disability issues from a theological and practical perspective."[46] Indeed, the program's report for the year 2002 was entitled "Creating Welcoming Congregations and Educating Clergy." Under the program, an outreach effort was initiated to seminaries in 2002 to "expose future religious leaders to both theological and practical issues of disabilities so their congregations will be tomorrow's welcoming houses of worship."[47] Several conferences had already been held "toward the goal of making seminaries more welcoming to faculty, staff, students, and visitors with disabilities."[48]

The initial conference for the "Seminary Project" was held on March 15, 2002 at Wesley Theological Seminary in Washington, D.C. The event was sponsored by Wesley Theological Seminary, N. O. D. and the Washington Theological Consortium and drew more than 100 participants from 14 theological schools. The Keynote Speaker, Dr. Nancy Eiesland of Candler School of Theology, Emory University, set the direction for the event by focusing on the point "that we are all created in the image of God," and that "seminaries are called upon to affirm that God's image takes many forms, not just one of bodily perfection."[49] Dr. Eiesland further stated that:

> Claiming disability means exploring the critical divisions our society makes in creating the normal versus the pathological, the insider versus the outsider, or the blessed versus the cursed. In the seminary context, claiming disability can provide new means for accessing faith, not only for people with disabilities, but for the entire community of faith.

She continued:

> The popular picture of the disabled life today encourages the view that people with disabilities constitute a perversion of God's creation. To counteract this perversion requires voices linguistically

sophisticated, intellectually nuanced and politically astute, capable of articulating the issues implicit in the full inclusion of people with disabilities in church and society.[50]

In one of five afternoon workshops, the Reverend Dr. Bruce C. Birch, Dean and Woodrow W. and Mildred B. Miller Professor of Biblical Theology at Wesley Theological Seminary, stated emphatically, that seminaries have a "'theological mandate' to address the issues of people with disabilities." In addition, Dean Birch stated:

> Whatever the nuances of our particular setting or tradition, theological schools are in the business of providing for the ministry of the whole people of God. If, on reflection, the disabled portion of God's people have been pushed to the margins, or left out altogether, then those of us who work and teach in seminaries have failed at our task.

> I would go further and say that it is also not enough to prepare those who would minister to the disabled in our communities, although sensitizing all in ministry to these issues is a worthy goal. We must be prepared to deal with the tough issues of preparing people with disabilities themselves for ministry so that ministry becomes by and with people with disabilities and not simply for them.[51]

Dean Birch outlined "four challenges facing seminaries as they strive to fully include, serve and serve with people with disabilities." The first was to provide the support services "necessary for students with disabilities to successfully complete the curriculum with integrity and participate in the formational life of the community." The second challenge was that of physical facilities. Seminaries should have a "plan with clear priorities for identifying and removing barriers," and that "adapting physical facilities extends beyond wheelchair access to include: [1] "Rearranging classrooms and reassigning courses to accessible classrooms, when necessary"; [2] "Providing special equipment, such as a small light in a darkened classroom to allow an ASL interpreter to be seen"; [and 3] "Signage indicating wheelchair accessible entrances and restrooms, and the offer of assistance where barriers have not yet been removed."[52]
The third and fourth challenges outlined were curriculum and faculty, respectively. According to Dean Birch, "issues of disability should

be addressed in courses throughout the curriculum. In addition, seminaries need to be alert to adjustments in the curriculum appropriate to students with disabilities. Traditional preaching courses, without adjustments, will be of little use to deaf students." Dean Birch, also indicated that "seminaries must also ask: [1] Do bibliographies include any of the rich literature now available? [and, 2] Do people with disabilities in the community serve as resources in classes?" He continued by indicating that:

> The faculty must be trained to develop sensitivities to issues facing people with disabilities. Ingrained habits, such as talking while facing the blackboard, are hard to change. Many of these issues are not obvious to people raised in environments that treat people with disabilities as either invisible or as somehow less able than others. Likewise, faculty must be careful not to assume what a student with a disability cannot do.[53]

The Conference concluded on a somber note acknowledging that "the challenges facing seminaries as they try to fully include and serve people with disabilities is no easy task." Among the limitations suggested by Dean Burch and others were the financial costs, the need for a critical student population (including the need to recruit qualified students with disabilities), and the need to recognize that some persons with disabilities may not have the skills to complete a seminary education. Nevertheless, the conference reaffirmed the call for "fully including people with disabilities in seminary life" as part of what Dr. Eiesland described as 'justice and just action.'" She emphasized that these are "primarily virtues and practices of full participation, of persons deliberating about particular visions of human flourishing and working together to remove barriers in their institutions and relations so that they embody reciprocity and mutual appreciation of difference." In addition:

> Justice demands equal access to safe and meaningful employment. The church must act in ways that witness this necessity. It must acknowledge in its educational and employment policies the gifts of people with disabilities and provide training, accommodations, and opportunities for those who are called by God to ministry and leadership.[54]

This one-day event served as the beginning of a major Religion and Disability Program thrust urging "seminaries to become welcoming and accessible to their members and visitors with disabilities." From this experience, the Seminary Project was formalized with stated goals and objectives. Its first goal is "to encourage seminaries to explore a range of theological and ethical issues with respect to people with disabilities." It is designed to confront a "theology that suggests disability is the result of sin or lack of faith" and replace it with "the view that children and adults with disabilities are created in the image of God." In addition, seminaries are encouraged to "provide opportunities for faculty, staff and students to negotiate tough spiritual, social justice, and ethical issues surrounding disability." The second goal is "to help seminaries welcome faculty, staff, students, and visitors with disabilities." This relates to the need for seminaries to provide such services as "regular awareness training" and the active recruitment of qualifies students with disabilities.

The third, and final, goal is "to better equip future religious leaders of America to serve and serve *with* children and adults with disabilities and their families." This ties the "Seminary Project" directly to the long-term efforts of the Religion and Disability Program. The objectives for this goal are as follows:

* Weave training and education on issues of disability throughout the curriculum. This includes core requirements and electives, field education, lecture series, and continuing education.
* Develop courses specifically focused on ministry with and for people with disabilities as a cross-cultural experience or requirement.
* Identify and assist family members of students, faculty, and staff who face issues of disabilities.
* Recruit faculty members, administrators, and staff with disabilities who can serve as role models.
* Give priority to internship sites and [field work] supervisors that offer rich contexts for sensitizing seminarians about issues of disability.
* Sponsor a "That All May Worship" conference on campus, fostering dialogue among disability advocates and their family members, seminary faculty and students, and religious leaders.[55]

Over the next few years, the Religion and Disability Program would encourage and help coordinate disability conferences and course offerings at a number of seminaries. In addition, the program would post numerous items on the N. O. D. website under the heading "Religious Participation (Seminaries: Access & Welcome)." Items included the full "goals" statement of the Seminary Project, summaries of the first conference (cited above), newspaper clippings and pictures from seminary "That All May Worship" conferences, and the N. O. D. Interfaith Directory of Religious Leaders with Disabilities. The Directory was created in 2001 as "a list of names and contact information for ordained clergy, religious educators, seminary faculty and seminarians with disabilities. The individuals on this list are willing to share their experiences with others in the religious community and disability communities."[56] The list currently has over 110 names posted on the N. O. D. website. The hope is that these leaders will be role models for others with disabilities who are considering seminary education.

The emphasis of the Religion and Disability Program is unique in that it is based in a secular organization (N. O. D.) and is available to religious leaders and people with disabilities of all faiths. Thus there is no distinctly Christian, Jewish, Muslim, or Buddhist way to offer hospitality to someone with disability. There is the universal way which is based on human dignity and respect. This interfaith vision is seen in several events occurring within the past few years.

The year 2003 witnessed the death of the Reverend Dr. Harold Wilke at the age of 88. As an N. O. D. Board Member and Founding Director, Wilke had served in numerous capacities and is credited with initiating the Religion and Disability Program in 1988. This was in keeping with his long career in four areas of service: the church, rehabilitation, teaching and government as well as his membership in the United Church of Christ, a denomination with a long history of working ecumenically and across faith lines. His commitment to both the secular and religious inclusion of people with disabilities is captured in his "blessing" given on July 26, 1990 at the White House bill signing of the American With Disabilities Act:

> Today we celebrate the breaking of the chains which have held back millions of Americans with disabilities. Today we celebrate the granting to them of full citizenship and access to the Promised Land of work, service and community.[57]

During 2003 and 2004, the Religion and Disability Program continued to thrive through its sale of publications, the Accessible Congregations Campaign, "That All May Worship" conferences and its outreach to theological schools. During 2003, "Director Ginny Thornburgh and her husband former Pennsylvania Governor Dick Thornburgh, received the 2003 Henry B. Betts Award honoring their contributions to the quality of life of people with disabilities." They and their son, Peter, are pictured in the *N. O.D. 2003 Annual Report* as Peter introduces them at the award ceremony.[58]

As 2005 approached, the Religion and Disability Program would continue to offer its full range of services. A record number of 25 "That All May Worship" conference were scheduled for the year and four seminaries (Princeton Theological Seminary, Luther Seminary, North American Baptist Seminary, and Auburn Theological Seminary) also scheduled disability conferences. The sale of its popular guides on religion and disability would contribute to sustaining the program, and the seventh updated version of "That All May Worship" was printed with funds from a two year grant from the W. H. Kellogg Foundation.[59] In addition, the Ramp brochure ("A Ramp is Not Enough") was reprinted with a grant from the Christopher Reeve Paralysis Foundation. On its website, N. O. D. paid tribute to Pope John Paul II (who died on April 2, 2005) as a "fellow advocate on behalf of the world's 600 million people with disabilities." From N. O. D.'s point of view:

> Pope John Paul II understood that people with disabilities have much to contribute, and late in his life, he led by example. He lived with Parkinson's disease and other health ailments, but feeling he still had work to do, he proceeded with his papal duties. Millions were inspired by his humanity and his drive. Though his hands shook, his speech was sometimes slurred and his infirmities increased in his later years, he pursued his mission and did not avoid appearing in public. His ailments were progressive, and he knew his own mortality, but he led on. In doing so, he gave a valuable lesson on the value of all life, young or old, with or without disability.[60]

It would also acknowledge, with pride, that in May, 2005, Ginny Thornburgh received the prestigious Hubert H. Humphrey Civil Rights Award presented by the Leadership Council on Civil Rights (LCCR) which celebrates "'outstanding individuals who best exemplify selfless and devoted service in the cause of equality,' and is widely seen as the civil rights community's highest honor."[61]

And so the Religion and Disability Program continues to add its interfaith voice to the on-going effort to integrate people with disabilities into every aspect of religious and community life. Perhaps the *2004*

N. O. D. Annual Report offers the best argument for both its success and continuing mission:

> Freedom of religion is one of the basic principles on which the United States was founded. However, for many people with disabilities, congregations are inaccessible and inhospitable. Barriers of architecture and attitude prevent people with disabilities from attending religious services as frequently as people without disabilities. Yet, as the Harris Survey results demonstrate, 84 percent of people with disabilities say their religious faith is important to them. Our goal is to ensure that people with and without disabilities who choose to worship, find a welcoming environment.[62]

NOTES

1. National Organization on Disability. *2001 Annual Report.* Washington, D.C. 2002. p. 3.
2. National Organization on Disability. *2001 Annual Report.* p. 2.
3. National Organization on Disability. *2001 Annual Report.* p. 2.
4. *Five Years of Progress: Toward Full Participation 1982-1986.* Washington, D.C., National Organization on Disability. (n.d.)
5. *Five Years of Progress: Toward Full Participation 1982-1986.*
6. *Toward Full Participation–The National Organization on Disability Annual Report for 1990.* Washington, D.C., National Organization on Disability, 1991
7. *Notes Prepared for Discussion with His Holiness Pope John Paul II.*
8. *Notes Prepared for Discussion with His Holiness Pope John Paul II.*
9. *Toward Full Participation–The National Organization on Disability Annual Report for 1990.*
10. *Toward Full Participation–The National Organization on Disability Annual Report for 1990.*
11. *National Organization on Disability: 1992 Annual Report.* Washington, D.C., National Organization on Disability.
12. *That All May Worship: An Interfaith Welcome to People with Disabilities.* Washington, D.C., The National Organization on Disability.
13. *National Organization on Disability: 1992 Annual Report.* National Organization on Disability, Washington, D.C.
14. *National Organization on Disability: 1993 Annual Report.* Washington, D.C., National Organization on Disability.
15. *National Organization on Disability: 1993 Annual Report.*
16. *National Organization on Disability: 1994 Annual Report.* Washington, D.C., National Organization on Disability.
17. *National Organization on Disability: 1994 Annual Report.*
18. *National Organization on Disability: 1994 Annual Report.*
19. *National Organization on Disability: 1994 Annual Report.*
20. *National Organization on Disability: 1995 Annual Report.*

21. *National Organization on Disability: 1995 Annual Report.*

22. *National Organization on Disability: 1996 Annual Report*, p. 19.

23. *N. O. D./Harris Survey of Americans with Disabilities.* 1994 The National Organization on Disability/Louis Harris and Associates, Inc., p. 136.

24. *N. O. D./Harris Survey of Americans with Disabilities.* 1994., p. 136.

25. *National Organization on Disability: 1996 Annual Report.*

26. *National Organization on Disability: 1996 Annual Report.*

27. *National Organization on Disability: 1996 Annual Report.*

28. *National Organization on Disability: 1996 Annual Report.*

29. *National Organization on Disability: 1997 Annual Report.*

30. *National Organization on Disability: 1998 Annual Report*, p. 11.

31. *National Organization on Disability: 1998 Annual Report*, p. 11.

32. *National Organization on Disability: 1998 Annual Report*, p. 11.

33. *The Accessible Congregations Campaign.* 1998. National Organization on Disability. Washington, D.C.

34. *The Accessible Congregations Campaign.* 1998.

35. *The Accessible Congregations Campaign.* 1998.

36. *National Organization on Disability: 1999 Annual Report*, p. 11.

37. *National Organization on Disability: 1999 Annual Report*, p. 11.

38. *National Organization on Disability: 1999 Annual Report*, p. 11.

39. *National Organization on Disability: 2000 Annual Report*, p. 13.

40. *National Organization on Disability: 2000 Annual Report*, p. 13.

41. *National Organization on Disability: 2001 Annual Report*, p. 1.

42. *National Organization on Disability: 2001 Annual Report*, p. 1.

43. *National Organization on Disability: 2001 Annual Report*, p. 1.

44. *National Organization on Disability: 2001 Annual Report*, p. 18.

45. *National Organization on Disability: 2001 Annual Report*, p. 18.

46. *National Organization on Disability: 2001 Annual Report*, p. 18.

47. *National Organization on Disability: 2002 Annual Report*, p. 8.

48. *National Organization on Disability: 2002 Annual Report*,. p. 8.

49. "Each Made in God's Image, Each a Unit of God's Grace." May, 2002. (A Summary of the Disability Convocation: Opening Heart, Minds and Doors in Seminary Communities, held at Wesley Theological Seminary on March 15, 2002.)

50. "Each Made in God's Image, Each a Unit of God's Grace." May, 2002.

51. "Each Made in God's Image, Each a Unit of God's Grace." May, 2002.

52. "Each Made in God's Image, Each a Unit of God's Grace." May, 2002.

53. "Each Made in God's Image, Each a Unit of God's Grace." May, 2002.

54. "Each Made in God's Image, Each a Unit of God's Grace." May, 2002.

55. "Goals: Seminary Project: Religion and Disability Program." National Organization on Disability. (n.d.)

56. "Religious Participation (Seminaries: Access & Welcome)." (See note 49)

57. *National Organization on Disability: 2003 Annual Report*, inside front cover.

58. *National Organization on Disability: 2003 Annual Report*, p. 12.

59. *National Organization on Disability: 2004 Annual Report*, p. 11.

60. "N. O. D. Pays Tribute to Pope John Paul II." National Organization on Disability, April 8, 2005.

61. "N. O. D.'s Ginny Thornburgh Receives Hubert H. Humphrey Civil Rights Award." *N. O. D. E-Newsletter, May 16, 2005.*

62. *National Organization on Disability: 2004 Annual Report.* p. 11.

Index